W9-BKA-661

Mayo Clinic Guide to Alzheimer's Disease

Ronald Petersen, M.D., Ph.D.

Medical Editor in Chief

Mayo Clinic
Rochester, Minnesota

Mayo Clinic Guide to Alzheimer's Disease provides reliable information about diagnosis, treatment and caregiving for Alzheimer's disease and other forms of dementia. This book supplements the advice of your personal physician, whom you should consult for individual medical problems. *Mayo Clinic Guide to Alzheimer's Disease* does not endorse any company or product. MAYO, MAYO CLINIC, MAYO CLINIC HEALTH SOLUTIONS and the Mayo triple-shield logo are marks of Mayo Foundation for Medical Education and Research.

Published by Mayo Clinic Health Solutions, Rochester, Minn. For bulk sales to employers, member groups and health-related companies, contact Mayo Clinic Health Solutions, 200 First St. S.W., Rochester, MN 55905, or send e-mail to SpecialSalesMayoBooks@Mayo.edu.

Photo credits: Cover photos and the photos on pages 1, 7, 76, 96, 113, 151, 171, 219, 246, 247, 253 and 255 are from PhotoDisc; photo on page 63 courtesy of the National Library of Medicine.

Library of Congress Catalog Card Number: 2005938465

ISBN-13: 978-1-893005-41-9
ISBN-10: 1-893005-41-0

Printed in Canada

First Edition

5 6 7 8 9 10

About Alzheimer's disease

Dementia is an umbrella term for many brain disorders that rob a person of memory and reason, and cause extreme changes to personality. These disorders generally are progressive and irreversible. Alzheimer's disease is the most common form of dementia. By 2050, a projected 13 million Americans will have Alzheimer's. Other forms of dementia include frontotemporal dementia, dementia with Lewy bodies and vascular cognitive impairment.

Although there is still no cure for Alzheimer's disease and no known strategies that prevent it, physicians are now able to diagnose the condition at much earlier stages and medications are available that may ease cognitive losses and greatly improve quality of life. Impressive advances in brain research over the last few decades offer real hope of providing answers to some of the most intractable mysteries surrounding the disease. It's hoped that with this new knowledge, more effective treatment and prevention of Alzheimer's disease will quickly follow.

About Mayo Clinic

Mayo Clinic evolved from the frontier practice of Dr. William Worrall Mayo and the partnership of his two sons, William J. and Charles H. Mayo, in the early 1900s. Pressed by the demands of their busy practice in Rochester, Minn., the Mayo brothers invited other physicians to join them, pioneering the private group practice of medicine. Today, with more than 2,000 physicians and scientists at its three major locations in Rochester, Minn., Jacksonville, Fla., and Scottsdale, Ariz., Mayo Clinic is dedicated to providing comprehensive diagnoses, accurate answers and effective treatments.

With this depth of medical knowledge, experience and expertise, Mayo Clinic occupies an unparalleled position as a health information resource. Since 1983, Mayo Clinic has published reliable health information for millions of consumers through award-winning newsletters, books and online services. Revenue from the publishing activities supports Mayo Clinic programs, including medical education and research.

Editorial staff

Medical Editor in Chief
Ronald Petersen, M.D., Ph.D.

Managing Editor
Kevin Kaufman

Publisher
Sara Gilliland

Editor in Chief, Books and Newsletters
Christopher Frye

Copyediting and proofreading
Miranda Attlesey
Mary Duerson
Louise Filipic
Linda Hager
Donna Hanson

Contributing Writers
Rachel Bartony
Lee Engfer
Jennifer Koski

Research Manager
Deirdre Herman

Research Librarians
Anthony Cook
Dana Gerberi
Michelle Hewlett

Creative Director
Daniel Brevick

Art Director
Stewart Koski

Illustration
Kent McDaniel

Medical Illustration
Michael King

Indexing
Steve Rath

Administrative Assistants
Beverly Steele
Terri Zanto-Strausbauch

Contributing editors and reviewers

Bradley Boeve, M.D.
Richard Caselli, M.D.
Dennis Dickson, M.D.
Daniel Drubach, M.D.
Yonas Geda, M.D.
Todd Golde, M.D.
Neill Graff-Radford, M.D.
Michael Hutton, Ph.D.
Robert Ivnik, Ph.D.
Clifford Jack, Jr., M.D.
Keith Josephs, M.D.

David Knopman, M.D.
Angela Lunde
Francine Parfitt
Joseph Parisi, M.D.
Maria Shiung
Glenn Smith, Ph.D.
Eric Tangalos, M.D.
Bryan Woodruff, M.D.
Karen Wallevand
Steven Younkin, M.D., Ph.D.

Preface

In 1906, Dr. Alois Alzheimer addressed an assembly of colleagues in Munich with his observations of an unusual brain disorder — a woman in her 50s affected by memory loss, confusion and hallucinations. This disorder subsequently came to bear his name and the publication of this book coincides with the 100th-year anniversary of Dr. Alzheimer's contribution.

Our knowledge of Alzheimer's disease has increased dramatically in the years since Dr. Alzheimer's report. Although it's still not possible to cure the disease, medications can ease its most distressing symptoms. An extensive network of resources supports Alzheimer's caregivers. Scientists are uncovering more about the complexities of the brain and revealing the causes and mechanisms of Alzheimer's that will ultimately lead to treatments that can delay or prevent the onset of this disorder. Of great significance is research on mild cognitive impairment, which represents the transition between a normally functioning brain and the initial stages of dementia. This early period offers the best hope for discovering an effective treatment for Alzheimer's. The book also addresses some of the less common but equally important forms of dementia.

Still, many older adults find themselves second-guessing every memory lapse and wondering if this isn't the start of dementia. One of the goals of this book is to help allay those fears. Although some of the changes brought on by aging affect brain function, Alzheimer's disease and the other forms of dementia described in this book are not part of normal aging. Millions of people age with their physical and mental health intact — and it's likely that you will too.

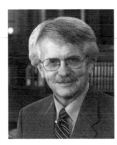

Ronald Petersen, M.D., Ph.D.
Medical Editor in Chief

Contents

Part 4: Expanding knowledge of dementia

Part 1

Aging and dementia

Many people worry that "growing old" includes memory loss, confusion and, possibly, a dementia such as Alzheimer's disease. These chapters explain what you may expect with age and they help you distinguish between normal and abnormal aging.

Chapter 1

What is dementia?

Hank is 80 years old, and proud to say that he has lived in the same house for 40 years. Though his wife died three years ago, he feels like he's doing OK on his own and doesn't need a lot of assistance from his family nearby. He has breakfast almost every morning in a neighborhood café, takes Rusty, his golden retriever, for a walk in the afternoons, and likes to tinker in his garage workshop. He's even learned to send e-mail on a computer that one of his children gave him. On the weekends, his grandchildren like to visit and help out a bit.

Some days, however, Hank forgets to feed Rusty in the morning, and on other days he forgets to feed himself lunch. On a few occasions, he's started out for the café, only to become confused about where he's going and had to return home. He's become moodier and less interested in socializing. He just can't seem to finish a workshop project anymore. The last time his grandchildren came over, he asked them what day of the week it was five times. On certain days, he insists that his wife is still alive.

Hank's children are concerned about the changes but Hank isn't concerned because Hank doesn't think there's a problem. Like many people who exhibit the signs and symptoms of cognitive decline, Hank doesn't recognize his own failing memory and troubling behavior.

Hank's story is an example of abnormal aging. Stiff joints, forgetfulness and gray hair are all signs of normal aging. But not all changes that occur later in life — changes often attributed to "aging" — are normal. These include severe memory loss, disorientation and personality changes that seriously impair a person's ability to perform routine activities and to interact socially. An individual may exhibit symptoms that suggest something may be wrong with brain function, and yet he or she is seemingly unaware of these problems. The person may be unable to formulate abstract thoughts, has difficulty carrying out simple tasks, is unable to control emotions and becomes easily agitated or paranoid.

Collectively, these signs and symptoms describe a syndrome called dementia. Dementia is a progressive mental disorder affecting millions of Americans.

What's a syndrome?

A syndrome is a collection of signs and symptoms that occur in a recognizable pattern to indicate a specific disease or condition. For example, the combination of severe memory loss, disorientation and personality change often leads to a diagnosis of dementia. It's important to stress that just memory loss (or disorientation or personality change) by itself doesn't mean dementia is present. It's the combination of signs and symptoms that's critical for a diagnosis.

Do you think that syndrome applies only to relatively rare conditions that will have little relevance to you? Guess again. For example, many women regularly experience headache, fatigue, breast tenderness and irritability before their menstrual cycles in what is known as premenstrual syndrome (PMS).

Many workers, especially those on an assembly line or who use a computer extensively, may be familiar with carpal tunnel syndrome, in which symptoms such as pain, tingling sensations in the hands and decreased grip strength define the condition. Well-known syndromes that have made recent headline news include acquired immunodeficiency syndrome (AIDS) and severe acute respiratory syndrome (SARS).

People with dementia don't just have mild memory lapses — they experience significant memory impairment that interferes with their ability to function in daily life. Other aspects of cognition are severely affected as well. The changes often happen gradually and secretively. Friends and family may be the first to notice one or more of the following signs and symptoms in their loved one:

- Having problems remembering recent events
- Repeatedly asking the same questions
- Becoming lost in familiar places
- Being unable to follow directions
- Being disoriented about time and place
- Being unable to handle personal finances
- Having problems finding the right word in conversations
- Neglecting personal safety, hygiene and nutrition

The term *dementia* isn't just another word for Alzheimer's disease. Rather, Alzheimer's is one of the most common causes of dementia. Dementia can be caused by many different disorders that affect the brain. Some of the symptoms above can be reversed with appropriate treatment, such as when the cognitive impairment is induced by high fever, drugs, dehydration or poor nutrition.

Most causes of dementia are irreversible, which means they cannot be cured and they grow progressively worse over time. These are often neurological disorders (of the central nervous system) or vascular disorders (of the circulatory system). Later chapters of this book are devoted to specific types of dementia.

Characteristics of dementia

In a general sense, dementia is the loss of various cognitive or intellectual functions that severely impairs your ability to function in daily life. This may involve memory loss, inability to use or understand language, inability to solve problems, loss of emotional control, personality changes and behavior problems, including delusions and hallucinations. The different types of dementia affect as many as 6.8 million Americans, and it's estimated that as many as 1.8 million of those people are severely affected.

Stages of dementia

The signs and symptoms of dementia vary considerably and no two people experience the disorder in the same way. That's partly because there are so many different and varied causes of dementia. An individual may be affected by some of the symptoms listed below or by many. The symptoms may be very subtle or very obvious.

Experts sometimes divide dementia into stages as a way to organize and describe the changes in the disease process in a logical and easily understood manner. Often, there are three stages designated as mild, moderate and severe.

Mild stage

One or more of the following signs and symptoms may develop in the early stages of dementia:

- Memory loss begins to affect abilities to function day to day
- Confusion and disorientation, especially in unfamiliar surroundings
- Poor judgment and decision making
- Mood and personality changes
- Loss of initiative to start tasks or projects
- Loss of spontaneity and enjoyment of life
- Trouble with calculations and handling finances
- More time required for routine tasks

Moderate stage

As dementia progresses, some of the following signs and symptoms may develop:

- Memory loss and confusion become more severe — along with a worsening of other signs and symptoms from the mild stage
- Shorter attention span and poor concentration
- Repetition, with physical movements or with statements and questions
- Restlessness and pacing

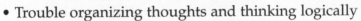

- Trouble organizing thoughts and thinking logically
- Inability to learn new information
- Problems communicating and using language
- Difficulty recognizing family and friends
- Periods of anxiety, irritation, paranoia or crying
- Behavior disorders, such as delusions and hallucinations
- Inability to control impulses
- Disrupted sleep
- Trouble with or neglect of personal care

Severe stage

In the late stages of dementia, the following signs and symptoms may develop:

- Worsening of symptoms from earlier stages of dementia
- Lack of self-awareness
- Loss of recent and remote memory
- Inability to recognize family and friends
- Inability to communicate verbally
- Dependence on others for personal care
- Weight loss
- Loss of bladder and bowel control
- Complications from infections, dehydration, seizures, pressure sores, swallowing and skin breakdown

These statistics may scare you — and lead you to believe that dementia is a common part of aging. But it's not. Only 4 percent to 8 percent of people over age 65 have moderate to severe dementia. The percentage goes up for people in their 80s — perhaps 30 percent of people of this age group have some form of dementia.

You may fear that you'll some day be part of these statistics and perhaps you're watching for the warning signs right now. Some of the most common signs and symptoms of dementia include:

- Severe memory loss
- Confusion and disorientation
- Problems with communication and language
- Persistently poor judgment
- Difficulty concentrating
- Inability to do things that used to be routine or come easily
- Difficulty carrying out complex or multiple tasks
- Inability to think abstractly
- Extreme personality changes and mood swings
- Inappropriate, bizarre or paranoid behavior

What causes these signs and symptoms? That's a question that scientists have been studying for decades. Because of the complexity of the human brain and the number of things that can go wrong, it's a difficult puzzle to solve. Many factors that can interfere with brain function are still unknown. But scientists do know that all forms of dementia result from the loss of communication between nerve cells and the deaths of these nerve cells.

A characteristic shared by certain dementing disorders such as Alzheimer's disease is the abnormal buildup of proteins in the brain. These proteins don't come from your diet but instead are produced by the body itself. Proteins are compounds that perform many vital tasks in your body — there are thousands of different kinds of proteins that do a thousand different things. Most scientists believe that the buildup of these proteins is toxic to neurons, and they suspect that it's at least one cause of the symptoms in people who have dementing disorders. Different proteins are associated with different disorders. Researchers are investigating ways to reduce, eliminate or prevent buildups in the hope that doing so may help treat the syndrome.

Another characteristic of certain types of dementia is the development of abnormal structures in the brain called inclusions. Certain kinds of inclusions are characteristic of certain kinds of dementia — for example, the deposits of alpha-synuclein protein in dementia with Lewy bodies — and it's suspected that they play a role in the development of symptoms. This issue is up for debate, however, with some scientists wondering if the inclusions are simply a side effect and not a cause of the disease process.

Primary causes of dementia

The many types of dementia are characterized by specific patterns of signs and symptoms. Sometimes these patterns are distinctive and sometimes they're subtle. Some types of dementia are caused by identifiable conditions and may be treatable. Other types have unknown causes and treatment can only ease the symptoms but not halt the disease process.

The most prevalent causes of dementia are neurodegenerative disorders and vascular disorders.

Neurodegenerative disorders

The term *neurodegenerative* may be a mouthful to say — but its meaning is fairly clear. Neurodegenerative disorders are those caused by the loss of or damage to neurons, or nerve cells, in the brain. There are four main types of neurodegenerative disorders that lead to dementia.

Alzheimer's disease. Alzheimer's disease is the most common cause of dementia, making up 50 percent to 60 percent of all cases of dementia. Alzheimer's disease is covered in great detail in Chapters 4 through 6.

People with Alzheimer's lose functioning neurons in areas of the brain associated with cognition and memory. In Alzheimer's early stages, those affected may experience memory loss and personality changes. As the disease progresses, memory and language problems worsen and difficulties with performing routine tasks becomes more common. Those affected may become disoriented,

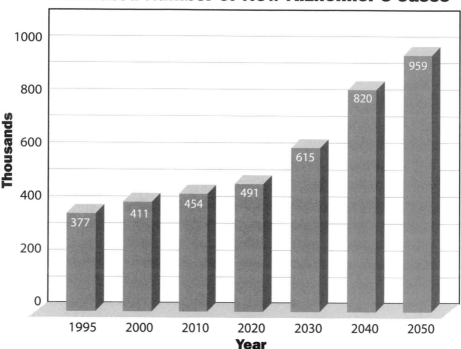

Estimated Number of New Alzheimer's Cases

The number of new cases of Alzheimer's disease reported each year is estimated to double over the next 50 years. By 2050, a projected 13 million people will have Alzheimer's disease in the United States.

delusional, and short-tempered or hostile. They may not recognize loved ones. Toward the end of the disease, basic functions — such as speaking, chewing and swallowing — may be seriously impaired or lost altogether.

Frontotemporal dementia. It's estimated that frontotemporal dementia (FTD) accounts for 2 percent to 10 percent of all cases of dementia. FTD refers to a group of brain disorders characterized by the loss of nerve cells in the frontal and temporal lobes of the brain. People with FTD experience behavior and personality disturbances. They may exhibit compulsive behavior, motor problems, and impaired speech and language. Although memory loss isn't usually a factor in the early stages, it does typically occur later in the disease. You can learn about frontotemporal dementia in Chapter 7.

Dementia with Lewy bodies. Dementia with Lewy bodies (DLB) gets its name from abnormal protein deposits, called Lewy

Causes of dementia

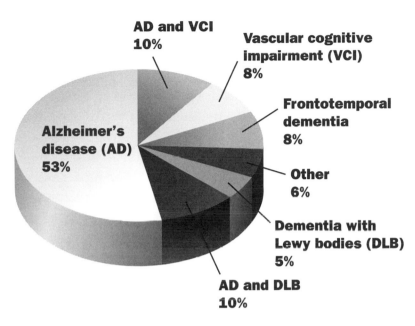

This pie is a rough approximation that gives you a general sense of dementia's many complex causes.

bodies, found in certain parts of the brain — specifically the cortex. Similar to Alzheimer's disease, signs and symptoms of dementia with Lewy bodies may include confusion, impaired memory, poor judgment and hallucinations. DLB may also mimic Parkinson's disease, with such symptoms as a shuffling, unsteady walk and bent posture. You can learn more about DLB in Chapter 8.

Parkinson's dementia. Parkinson's disease is a degenerative disorder that causes tremors and muscle stiffness. People in late stages of the disease may develop dementia, but this is not always the case.

Vascular disorders

Your vascular system involves the heart, arteries and veins that circulate blood through your body — from your head to your feet and everywhere in between. Conditions such as cardiovascular disease, high blood pressure and atherosclerosis compromise the health of your vascular system, putting you at risk for several types of vascular disorders. Dementia that can be caused by a vascular disorder is known as vascular cognitive impairment (VCI).

One of the most common forms of vascular cognitive impairment is caused by a series of small strokes to the brain. These strokes typically cause multiple areas of damaged tissue, called infarcts, and result in lesions in the brain's white matter.

Unlike Alzheimer's disease, the onset of vascular cognitive impairment may be sudden if the strokes are severe and may progress in step-by-step fashion with additional strokes. These symptoms may include cognitive loss, decreased motor skills, and delusions or depression. Depending on the locations of the infarcts, symptoms may be limited to one side of the body or just one or two specific functions may be affected. Although damage to brain tissue cannot be reversed, factors that increase the chance of future strokes — such as high blood pressure or cardiovascular disease — can be treated, helping to prevent further damage. You can learn more about VCI in Chapter 9.

Diagnosing a specific cause of dementia isn't as easy as checking off items on a list. The various causes — both neurodegenerative and vascular — may share common signs and symptoms. Frequently, two types of dementia occur at the same time, making it difficult to distinguish between them.

For example, memory loss and confusion are two of the most characteristic symptoms of both Alzheimer's disease and dementia with Lewy bodies. Lewy body inclusions also can be found in the brains of people with Parkinson's disease. Scientists continue to study whether DLB is simply related to other causes of dementia such as Alzheimer's or Parkinson's, or if these are different types of dementia that can coexist in the same person. These research efforts should hopefully make diagnosis easier in the future.

Other causes of dementia

Other conditions may cause dementia or dementia-like symptoms. Some of these you may have heard of, or even experienced, without being aware that dementia could result. What distinguishes

Is it a cause or a type of dementia?

You may hear a condition such as Alzheimer's disease referred to as a cause of dementia in one instance and a type of dementia in the next. Sound a little confusing? Both designations are correct — it all depends on what a physician has learned about the condition at a particular point in the disease process.

Physicians evaluate signs and symptoms at the initial office visit without necessarily knowing their cause. If the results of this evaluation best fit the criteria for Alzheimer's disease, the physician will say that Alzheimer's is the likely *cause* of the dementia.

Once Alzheimer's disease has been identified clinically as the cause, however, there's a transition in how it's designated. The *type* of dementia is known from now on as Alzheimer's disease — or, more specifically, "dementia of the Alzheimer type."

some of these causes is the fact that the dementia may be reversible — meaning it can be cured — with the proper treatment.

Some infectious diseases, for example, can cause dementia-like symptoms as your body works to overcome the infection. Infections that occur in the brain, such as meningitis, may also cause confusion, impaired judgment and memory loss. However, when caught early, both the infection and resulting dementia can be cured when treated properly. This is why it's so important to talk with your doctor if you're experiencing problems with your memory and concentration. More detail on these causes of dementia can be found in Chapter 10.

Besides the primary causes described earlier in this chapter, other causes of dementia include:

Infection. The inflammation of brain structures from infections such as meningitis and encephalitis can damage brain cells.

Reaction to medication. The side effects from some drugs can cause temporary problems with memory and concentration.

Metabolic or endocrine imbalances. Diseases of the thyroid, kidney, pancreas and liver can upset the chemical balance in your blood, causing delirium or dementia.

Normal pressure hydrocephalus. When cerebrospinal fluid builds up in the ventricles of the brain, the brain tissue is compressed even though the fluid pressure remains normal.

Brain tumors. Certain tumors may cause dementia symptoms, for example, if they press against brain structures that control hormone levels.

Subdural hematoma. Blood collecting beneath the outer covering of the brain can cause dementia-like symptoms.

Heart and lung problems. Conditions such as heart disease, emphysema and pneumonia can deprive the blood stream of oxygen, causing cell death and possibly dementia.

Nutritional deficiencies. Deficiencies of certain nutrients, such as the B vitamins, may cause the symptoms of dementia.

Chronic alcoholism. Dementia may result from the complications of chronic alcoholism, such as liver disease and nutritional deficiencies.

Substance abuse. Misuse of prescription drugs, such as sleeping pills and tranquilizers, may cause dementia symptoms. Street drugs, especially in high doses, can have a similar effect.

Poisoning. Exposure to toxic solvents or fumes without protective equipment can damage brain cells and lead to dementia.

Cognitive problems that aren't dementia

Sometimes you may worry that a loved one is showing signs and symptoms of dementia, when it's really nothing of the sort. For instance, mild memory loss is common as you grow older. While some people fear this decline is the first step to dementia, it's more often a slowing down of your mental processing and, with some accommodation for the forgetfulness, little cause for alarm.

A more serious form of memory loss is associated with mild cognitive impairment (MCI). This condition occurs when people experience cognitive problems beyond what's considered normal, age-related decline — but not so much that their quality of life or ability to perform daily activities is impaired. Though MCI isn't severe enough to be considered dementia, people who experience it do have a significantly increased risk of developing dementia in the future. For more on MCI, see Chapter 11.

Two other conditions — depression and delirium — may also mimic dementia. Although these conditions exhibit some of the same signs and symptoms as dementia, they're both treatable.

Depression

In the most general sense, the term *depression* describes a temporary low mood that comes from a bad day or a bad feeling. But as a medical term, depression denotes a serious illness that affects your thoughts, emotions, feelings, behaviors and physical health. People used to think it was "all in your head" and that if you really tried, you could pull out of the mood. Doctors now know that depression is not a weakness and you can't treat it on your own. It's a medical disorder with a biological or chemical basis.

Sometimes, a stressful life event triggers depression, such as retirement or the death of a spouse. Other times depression seems to occur spontaneously with no identifiable cause. Regardless, depression is much more than grieving or a bout of the blues.

Like those who experience dementia, people with depression may be confused, forgetful and slow to respond. The condition affects how they feel, think, eat, sleep and act in everyday life. Two hallmark symptoms of depression are an ongoing sense of sadness and despair and an inability to enjoy normal daily activities that once brought pleasure.

Although it may be difficult to know if a person is depressed, you might look for some of the following signs:

- Unexplained weight loss or gain — and, accordingly, reduced or increased appetite
- Sleep disturbance
- Irritability and anxiety
- Agitated behavior and restlessness
- Fatigue
- Lack of energy and initiative
- Poor concentration
- Feelings of low self-esteem
- Thoughts of death

If the person seems easily distressed and he or she wasn't that way before, that also might be a sign of depression. If you observe any of these changes, inform your doctor. Even if the symptoms aren't associated with depression, it's important to identify any underlying reasons for distress, such as physical discomfort.

Medications are available that are generally safe and effective, such as antidepressants and mood-stabilizing drugs. With proper treatment, most people with serious depression will improve.

Depression is the most common condition that accompanies various types of dementia. You would expect brief periods of discouragement and apathy to develop when someone is dealing with a serious disorder, but prolonged despondency should not be left untreated. On occasions when dementia is also present, the negative impact of depression on your emotions and intellect can be more extreme. For more about depression and Alzheimer's disease, see pages 75-76 in Chapter 4.

Delirium

Delirium is a state of mental confusion, disordered speech and clouded consciousness. Those affected may be disoriented and going through a range of personality changes. Though these signs and symptoms may be mistaken for those of dementia, there are important differences.

One difference is the abruptness with which the signs and symptoms of delirium develop. Someone who exhibits sudden disorientation, agitation, loss of consciousness or hallucinations is more likely to have delirium than dementia.

Another difference is that delirium is often caused by a treatable physical or psychiatric illness. In such cases, emergency medical treatment of delirium is vital because the underlying cause may be a serious illness such as bacterial meningitis. Delirium can be common in older adults who have lung or heart disease, long-term infections, poor nutrition, medication interactions or hormone disorders. Someone with dementia also can develop delirium, often from a complication such as a urinary tract infection.

The point to remember is that whether depression and delirium occur alone or in combination with dementia, both are treatable conditions. If you or a loved one may be exhibiting signs and symptoms of either, plan to see a doctor. The sooner the condition is diagnosed, the sooner you may find relief and start to feel better.

Risk factors for dementia

What can put you at risk of dementia? There's a range of factors, actually. Some, such as age and family history, are unavoidable and cannot be changed. Others, however, are lifestyle related, which means you can minimize their impact — or avoid them altogether.

As you read the list below, remember that having several of these risk factors doesn't mean that dementia is foretold in your future. Calculating risk can be an inexact science — it's an estimate of your chances of getting a disease over a certain period of time — and by no means is it definitive.

Age. The risk of getting dementia goes up significantly with advancing age. While only 4 percent to 8 percent of people over age 65 have dementia, for instance, over 30 percent of people in their 80s are thought to have some form of the disease.

Genes. Researchers have identified a number of genes and gene mutations that increase the risk of developing a dementia. As a rule, for example, people with a family history of Alzheimer's disease are considered to have a higher risk of developing the disease than people without a family history. Research suggests that risk may be two to three times higher if a parent or sibling has the disease. Of course, rules are made to be broken — and many people with a family history of the disease never develop Alzheimer's. The bottom line is that it's still not possible to predict an individual's risk of dementia strictly based on genetic evidence.

Atherosclerosis. The risk of vascular cognitive impairment increases with the presence of atherosclerosis, a buildup of cholesterol and fatty deposits on artery walls, which interferes with the delivery of blood to the brain and can lead to stroke.

High cholesterol. Like atherosclerosis, high levels of low-density lipoprotein (LDL, or "bad cholesterol") significantly increase a person's risk of developing vascular cognitive impairment.

Diabetes. Diabetes can damage blood vessels in the brain and increase the risk of vascular cognitive impairment. In addition, ongoing research is uncovering possible links between diabetes and Alzheimer's disease.

Smoking. Although somewhat controversial, some experts believe that people who smoke have a significantly higher risk of dementia. That's because smokers have a higher risk of atherosclerosis and other types of vascular disease. These conditions, in turn, increase the risk of dementia.

Alcohol use. Drinking large amounts of alcohol on a regular basis increases the risk of dementia.

Assessing the changes

What becomes a key issue as you grow older is your willingness to accommodate the changes brought on by the aging process while still maintaining your quality of life — you try to adapt to changes but at what price? If you carry one or more of the risk factors for dementia, you may be that much more concerned.

Take time to assess how you're dealing with growing old. Chapter 2 can provide more information on what to expect with normal aging. Also depend on your own judgment, intuition and experience. It's not always easy to distinguish between normal and abnormal changes. Often, the differentiation is a slight matter of degree. Do you occasionally forget an appointment or misplace your keys, or are the memory problems a daily experience that frustrate you?

Focus on the disruption that these changes bring to your daily life. If you feel that your routines have become too disordered and you're unable to perform simple tasks as you did before, these may not be normal changes you're experiencing. You may need to take the initiative and consider contacting your doctor for an evaluation.

Chapter 2

What to expect as you grow older

Mary feels healthy. The 62-year-old grandmother of five eats well, takes daily walks and tends a beautiful garden. She lives in her own home, and prides herself on her independence. But lately, she's noticing that her memory isn't what it used to be. She's been misplacing items, such as her purse and car keys. She forgot a doctor appointment last week, and when she came out of the drugstore this morning she couldn't remember where she parked her car. She worries that if memory slips such as these continue her independent life will end.

John, 67, lives with his wife of 45 years in an apartment complex for seniors. He enjoys doing crossword puzzles, meeting with his morning coffee group, and visiting his children across the country. A former college professor, he's always considered his mind to be "sharp." But lately John has noticed that, even though he continues to read extensively and listen to news, his recall of facts has diminished sharply. Sometimes, in conversations, he leaves a thought hanging in midsentence as he struggles to find the right word. For John, losing the ability to discuss topics that interest him will threaten a good bit of the joy he takes in life.

Although Mary and John haven't discussed their concerns with anyone yet, they both fear that these mental lapses could be leading to something more serious: Alzheimer's disease.

Alzheimer's disease (AD), the most common cause of age-related dementia, is a fear of many adults as they grow older. Some imagine contracting the disease as probable, while others consider it an inescapable fate. In almost any community, you can find someone who's providing care for a parent, sibling or friend who has dementia. You regularly read or hear headline reports about Alzheimer's in newspapers, television and radio. It's no wonder then, if you're over age 60, that you may find yourself second-guessing minor memory lapses and wondering if these aren't the first signs of the disease.

Addressing a common question

More people are reaching their "golden years" in America than ever before. In 2003, average life expectancy rose to its highest level yet at 77.6 years. That's 30 years longer than Americans were expected to live just 100 years ago. The trend doesn't appear to be slowing down. While approximately 36 million Americans are over age 65 today, the U.S. Census Bureau projects that 86.7 million people will be in this age group by 2050.

This chapter addresses the common question of just about any individual facing old age: Am I getting Alzheimer's? How do you distinguish between the changes in your body that are simply due to aging and those that could signal a potentially serious problem such as dementia?

It may be best to start by understanding what "healthy aging" means. There are indeed a number of changes — memory loss included — that commonly occur as you age. Many of your physical capabilities diminish and thinking skills naturally slow down. Those changes are described in this chapter.

Being familiar with the normal process of aging may allay most of your initial fears — and it can increase your awareness and guide your response should a potential problem develop. Later chapters in this book are devoted to specific forms of dementia, such as Alzheimer's disease, as well as practical guidelines for caregiving to someone who has dementia.

How long will you live?

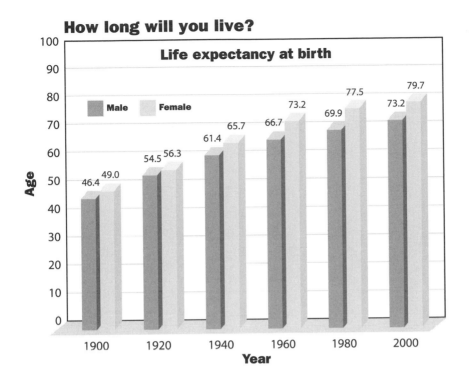

Timing, as they say, is everything. If you were a baby in 1900, you could expect to reach your mid- to late 40s. If you survived the onslaught of childhood diseases and you reached age 65, you'd probably live until your mid-70s. On the other hand, if you were born in 2000 and you live to age 65, you can expect to live until your early to mid-80s.

Source: Office of the Chief Actuary, Social Security Administration

Rest assured, however, that many conditions and diseases often associated with growing older, such as Alzheimer's disease, are not normal. Millions of people age with their physical and mental health intact — and it's likely that you will, too.

Physical changes with normal aging

Regardless of how well you live, the wear and tear of time takes a toll on the organs and systems in your body. You probably started noticing this as early as your 30s and 40s, when it became just a little bit harder to bounce back from a cold or keep up a vigorous pace when you exercised.

Defining normal

How do people typically age? When it comes to changes in cognitive function, what's normal — and what may be cause for concern? You might be surprised to learn that research into normal aging has lagged behind studies of cognitive abnormality and dementia. One reason is that although most people assume they know what's normal, the answer isn't always as straightforward as it might seem.

For example, does "normal" apply to the centenarian who still lives in her own home, walks her dog every day, plays bingo twice a week, and whose mind is as sharp as ever? We know people like this exist, but they're usually few and far between. This is the type of aging that most people ideally want to experience, but it's certainly not normal in terms of numbers. Experts refer to cases such as this, where there is little cognitive decline over time, as successful aging or optimal aging.

More often, aging is accompanied by illnesses and conditions such as heart disease, high blood pressure, and the loss of hearing and vision. Although the effects of these conditions on cognitive health is still uncertain, most people do experience slight forgetfulness and slower reaction times with age. Such changes are viewed as common parts of aging, even though they may be caused by disease. They may be inconvenient and frustrating but aren't debilitating — a person can still live an active, independent life in spite of the problems. This experience may be referred to as typical aging.

The challenge lies in distinguishing typical aging from abnormal changes that signal the beginnings of dementia. In studying and defining the earliest stages of the disorder, scientists hope to capture dementia when it's most amenable to treatment. At the same time, brain experts are also exploring the concept of successful aging, what it means and what can be done to promote lifelong mental health. Both tracks of research will provide valuable insight into the prevention of cognitive decline. (For more information on successful aging, see Chapter 11 on staying mentally sharp.)

Some of the physical changes of aging, such as graying or thinning hair, are visible to the world around you. Your skin may become thinner, drier and less elastic, causing it to wrinkle and sag. You may bruise more easily, and age spots may begin to appear.

Other changes are less noticeable to others. Your mouth may feel drier. The walls of your bladder become less elastic so you have to go to the bathroom more often. Because your breathing capacity declines, vigorous exercise may be more difficult.

Some age-related changes are so subtle that you may not even notice them. For instance, your digestive system slows and your immune system is less effective. Kidney function declines, so you're more likely either to become dehydrated or to retain fluid.

For many people, these changes may not cause serious difficulties. Other age-related physical changes, however, may be more troubling. Some may increase your risk of dementia or be mistaken as a symptom of dementia.

Cardiovascular changes

A healthy cardiovascular system is key to the well being of every organ in your body — and that includes your brain. Comprised of the heart and an intricate network of blood vessels, the cardiovascular system delivers nutrients and oxygen to body tissues and removes waste products from them

With age, your heart muscle becomes less efficient, working harder to pump the same amount of blood through your body. By age 60, about 35 percent less blood circulates through the arteries of the heart (coronary arteries) than in earlier years.

In addition, arteries tend to thicken and become stiff with age, further increasing the amount of work your heart must do to pump blood. Over time, fatty deposits may accumulate in the artery walls, narrowing the passageway through these vessels.

Despite the changes, an older heart can still function well. At rest, the differences between younger and older hearts are minor. Most people can maintain a fairly active life — trouble occurs primarily when sudden demands are placed on the aging heart. And it takes longer for the heart rate and blood pressure to return to normal levels after a stressful event.

Although most age-related changes in the cardiovascular system don't affect everyday functioning, an older person is at higher risk of high blood pressure, coronary artery disease and congestive heart failure. An older individual is also at greater risk of stroke. Such vascular disorders may increase your risk for dementia.

Skeletal and muscular changes

As you get older, your bones shrink in size and in density. In addition, the gel-like disks that cushion the vertebrae of your spine become thinner. Muscle mass tends to decrease, and joints and tendons lose some strength and flexibility. Movement often slows and becomes more limited as you age, which may be frustrating for some. Balance and coordination diminish, greatly increasing your risk of falls. Still, most people find that their muscles and bones remain strong enough to allow them to perform daily tasks.

Sensory changes

Changes to vision and hearing can be especially troubling as you age, making it more difficult to communicate or do the things you used to enjoy. If these changes go undetected, they can result in inappropriate actions that others may misinterpret as dementia.

Vision. Changes to your eyesight are often some of the first signs of aging. By age 55, almost everyone will need glasses, at least part of the time, to correct refractive problems. With age, you're more at risk of eye disorders such as cataracts, glaucoma and age-related macular degeneration.

Hearing. About one-third of Americans over age 60 and half of all people over age 85 have hearing problems. Hearing loss may result from damage to structures of the inner ear or to hearing pathways of the outer ear. Many things can contribute to hearing loss, including a buildup of earwax, exposure to loud noises, certain medications, head injuries and illnesses.

Metabolism changes

With age, your metabolism generally slows down. Metabolism involves thousands of chemical processes that regulate many body functions. Many of the changes associated with aging are a result of changes to this system. With age, growth hormones and sex hormones decrease, and you burn fewer calories than you once did, making it harder to lose weight. Not all hormones decrease with age, however. Some remain unchanged, while others increase. And some of these changes may increase your risk of dementia.

Your brain and how it works

Not surprisingly, the aging process brings changes to your brain. Weighing in at about three pounds, the brain is the most complex, amazing organ in your body. Think of it as your very own master computer. The brain controls actions you think about, such as balancing the checkbook or debating political views, along with actions you don't think about, such as swallowing food, regulating heartbeat or blinking dust from your eye.

In a normal, healthy state, the brain manages vital body functions and physical actions. It directs basic instincts, memory, intellectual analysis and creative thought. It organizes and shapes emotions. Most miraculously, perhaps, the brain enables you to do many of these things at the same time.

Consider something as simple as reading a book. In addition to absorbing the meaning of the words, you're likely holding the book upright, adjusting the distance from your eyes for clear vision and turning pages at the appropriate times. You're analyzing the story as it's being read, as well as processing sounds and sensations in the environment around you, keeping an eye on the clock — and maybe sipping from your coffee cup. Your brain controls all of these actions. Simultaneously, your brain is managing vital functions of survival — breathing air, pumping blood, maintaining body temperature and digesting food.

Functional tour of the brain

Your brain is made up of distinct structures, with each structure performing a variety of specific tasks. These structures include:

Brain stem. Located at the base of your brain, the brain stem is responsible for some of the most basic functions you need to survive, including breathing, digesting food and controlling heart rate. It also connects the rest of your brain to your spinal cord.

Cerebellum. The cerebellum, which sits at the back of the brain stem, is responsible for balance, movement and coordination. The cerebellum helps you do such things as stand upright, walk from one room to another and ride a bike.

Cerebrum. While the brain stem and cerebellum are busy handling the many involuntary actions and adjustments in your body, your cerebrum performs the "thinking" functions of your brain. It's responsible for a large part of who you are as an individual.

Resting on top of the brain stem, the cerebrum is the largest structure of the human brain and probably the most recognizable. To get a rough picture of what your cerebrum looks like, make two fists and put them together in front of you. Like your left and right fists, your cerebrum is divided into left and right hemispheres separated by a deep groove. These two hemispheres are connected by a thick band of nerve cell fibers called the corpus callosum.

Each hemisphere of the brain is comprised of four lobes, with each lobe responsible for different functions. For example, the

Lobes of the brain

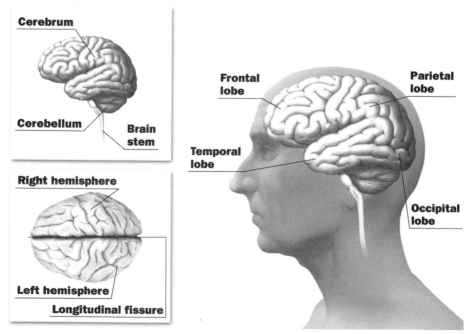

frontal lobe in each hemisphere is associated with personality, problem solving, abstract thought and skilled movement.

Behind the frontal lobe in each hemisphere is the parietal lobe, which handles sensory information such as pain, taste and touch. This lobe supports your visuospatial abilities, those abilities that allow you to navigate your surroundings without bumping into objects or to assemble the interlocking pieces of a jigsaw puzzle.

The temporal lobe is situated at the side of the forehead, roughly at the location of your temple. It's vital for hearing and language comprehension and is involved with perception and memory.

At the back of each hemisphere is the occipital lobe. You may have heard this lobe called by another name, the visual cortex, since it's primarily responsible for your vision.

The outer surface of your cerebrum is a layer of tissue less than a quarter of an inch thick. Grayish-brown and wrinkled looking, this layer is called the cerebral cortex — though you may also have heard it called gray matter. The cerebral cortex is where most of your intellectual operations — thinking, reasoning, analyzing,

The functional brain

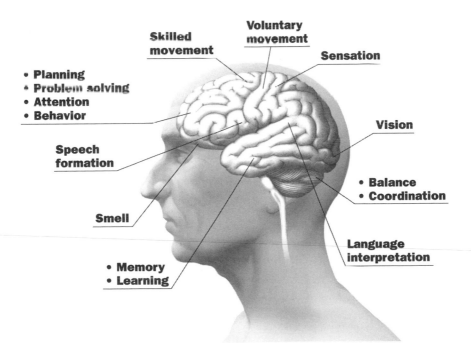

organizing, creating, decision making and planning — take place. The grooves and folds of the cortex allow a greater surface area to fit inside the skull, thus increasing the amount of information that can be processed. Underneath the cerebral cortex is white matter, which plays an important role in the transmission of nerve impulses to and from the various structures of your brain.

Limbic system. The limbic system is comprised of several small structures located in the internal regions of the brain and associated with your emotions and sense of motivation. Its job is to sort through the millions of sensory messages bombarding your brain and to regulate vital body systems. The limbic system includes:

Hypothalamus. The hypothalamus (hi-po-THAL-uh-muhs) sits near the center of your brain, and controls body functions such as eating, sleeping and sexual behavior. It maintains chemical balance and regulates hormones. It also controls your body temperature — telling your body, for example, to sweat if you're too hot and to shiver if you're too cold.

Amygdala. The amygdala (uh-MIG-duh-luh) governs such emotions as anger and fear and triggers your response to danger, whether that response is confronting a situation or fleeing it (commonly called the fight-or-flight response). You call the amygdala to action, for example, when you see a strange dog approaching and you decide whether to run, reach out to it or call for help.

Hippocampus. The hippocampus (hip-o-KAM-pus) plays a crucial role in your memory system. It's responsible for sorting new pieces of information, storing them in the appropriate parts of your brain and recalling them when necessary. It acts as your brain's switchboard — transferring information between your recent and remote memories — and helps you remember everything, from where you left your car keys this morning to where you vacationed in the summer as a child.

Thalamus. Another internal structure of the brain, separate from the limbic system, is the thalamus. The job of the thalamus is to process information from your senses, and then transmit this information to other parts of your brain.

In a normal, healthy brain, all of these structures work together in a remarkably efficient, coordinated fashion. They're protected by the bony shell of your skull and cushioned by layers of membrane. An intricate network of blood vessels supplies the food and oxygen they need in order to function.

The brain and spinal cord make up your central nervous system. Extending from your spinal cord is a network of nerves that branch out through your body, all the way to the tips of your fingers and toes. This network is called the peripheral nervous system. These nerves are continually gathering sensory information from inside and outside your body and relaying messages to your brain.

Your brain can receive hundreds of these messages in an instant. As your

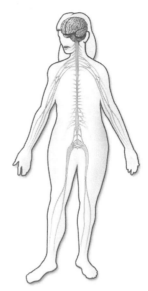

Nervous system

brain interprets the messages, relevant bits of information are sent to different parts of your brain for memory storage. When interpretation — which can be a split-second process — is complete, the brain shoots back instructions that tell your fingers, legs, mouth, heart or any other part of your body how to respond.

By rapidly processing, sorting, filing and responding to this continuous barrage of incoming messages, your brain gives meaning to the world around you. The manner in which your brain performs these tasks, which is different from the way any other person's brain functions, makes you the unique person you are.

Cell communication

Your brain's nerve cells are called neurons — and you have about 100 billion of them. These neurons are the basic units of your brain and nervous system. They allow different parts of your body to communicate by generating electric impulses, or messages.

Each neuron is designed to collect and process messages, then relay the information to other cells. The cell body, called the soma, contains the nucleus and other structures. Branching out from the cell body are fibers called dendrites. The dendrites' job is to receive messages from adjoining nerve cells.

A single branch called an axon, larger than a dendrite, also extends out from the cell body. The axon carries messages away from the neuron, so that it can relay these messages to other cells. Linked from axon to dendrite, neurons form continuous pathways that messages follow to any part of the body.

Wrapped around most axons is a fatty substance called myelin. Myelin helps insulate the axon and speeds up the transmission of messages. Myelin-covered axons, which appear white, are found in the white matter of the cerebrum.

In order for a neuron to send a message, something must spur it into action. This can range from a prick on your finger to a funny scene in a movie to a relayed message from another neuron. When this happens, an electric impulse travels like a wave through the neuron's cell body to the tip of the axon. There it encounters neuro-transmitters — tiny sacs of chemicals that act as data messengers. When the impulse arrives, it signals the release of these neurotrans-mitters into a synapse, which is the space between the axon and an

Neuron structure

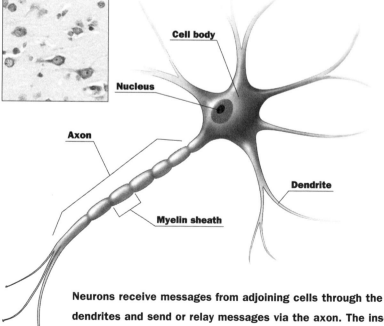

Neurons receive messages from adjoining cells through the dendrites and send or relay messages via the axon. The inset at upper left is a microphotograph that shows neurons in brain tissue.

adjoining cell. In the synapse, the neurotransmitters make a path to receptors on the receiving cell. The membrane of the receiving cell is then altered in a way that re-creates the impulse, and the process begins again in the next neuron.

In this way, a message is passed from neuron to neuron until the impulse travels to its intended destination, which could be a part of the brain, an organ such as your heart or any one of your muscles.

In simple terms, think of this process as an incredibly accurate game of "telephone" that children often play. One child whispers a message into the ear of the next child, who turns to whisper the message into the next child's ear, and so on until an entire line of children has received the message — and can now act on it together. Only, in your brain, this process happens in lightning-fast speed, and the message doesn't get garbled along the way.

Making memories

Memory involves your ability to store, recall and reuse the information you take in. You might think that your brain is like a library filled with rooms of shelved books — or, in this case, memories — just waiting to be checked out and read. But this analogy is only half true. Because, unlike a library, your brain doesn't store an entire memory on a single shelf. Instead, the part of your brain called the hippocampus breaks memories down into smaller pieces — such as how an object looks, smells, sounds and feels — then stores these individual pieces in different parts of your brain.

For example, the melody of a favorite song may be stored in your temporal lobes, the areas of your brain that allows you to interpret sounds. The song's lyrics, on the other hand, may be stored in different areas of your frontal and parietal lobes. Certain emotions that you always associate with this song or information that you know about the singer may be shelved in other parts of your brain. So, whenever the song comes on the radio, your brain reassembles its memory from many different locations — and, there you have it — you can sing along.

Your brain functions with two different kinds of memories: recent and remote. Your recent memory is for information that you need to remember for, well, short amounts of time. It's what you use for that 30-second interval between the time you look up a number in the phone book and the time you dial the phone. Recent memory has a high "turnover rate," meaning information is continually replaced with newer information. Recent memory helps keep your brain clutter-free, allowing you to discard numbers and facts that you don't need.

Remote memory, on the other hand, is designed to be stored in your brain for longer amounts of time so that you can access this information when you need it — whether in 10 hours or 10 years. Your remote memory retains your computer password, the direc-

How memory works

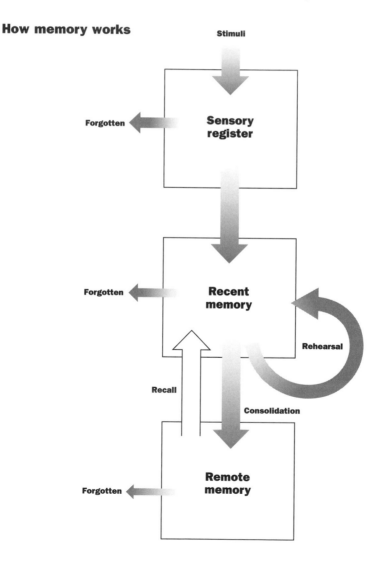

tions to a friend's house, and how you got that scar on your knee when you were 12 years old.

For a memory to become remote, it must go through a process called consolidation. When you learn information, such as the name of your new neighbor, it forms a neural pathway in your brain. For that information to become a part of your long-term memory, the pathway must be strengthened. How does this happen? By focusing your attention on the information when you first learn it, by repeating or rehearsing the information often, or by associating the information with more familiar knowledge.

Say you're learning to play the piano. You strike a skinny black key and the sound of it vibrates briefly in your ears. That brief millisecond of recognition is your sensory register in action. Then your teacher points to a squiggle on a piece of paper in front of you and says, "That's the note for an E flat." You hit the key again. The sound of the note and the information you received from your teacher are now registered in your recent memory.

If you go away and never play that note again, the information you learned will likely be forgotten and you will probably not remember what an E flat sounds like. If, however, you practice regularly, associating the note on the paper with the key you're playing, this information will pass into your remote memory.

Emotionally charged events can also be registered in your remote memory, although they don't need the repetition of learned information. Do you remember what you were doing when the World Trade Center and the Pentagon were attacked on Sept. 11, 2001? Many people vividly remember where they were and what they were doing at the instant of a calamity.

Cognitive changes with normal aging

Starting around age 50, many people begin to notice cognitive changes that directly affect memory and other brain functions. As you age, the number of neurons in your brain decreases and the number of connections between nerve cells is reduced. As a result, your brain atrophies, or "shrinks," as brain mass decreases.

What is cognition?

The term *cognition* comes from the Latin word *cognoscere*, which means "to know." It refers to all processes of the brain that allow you to think and consciously act, to interact with and experience your surroundings, and to feel emotions. The mental processes of "knowing" involve awareness, perception, judgment, reason, learning and memory. Cognitive processes are in contrast to many involuntary or unconscious processes that your body undertakes to function, such as the regulation of heartbeat and respiration.

These changes may sound foreboding, but they're really not. With billions of neurons and trillions of connections between them, the brain has a much greater capacity than is required for normal needs in a lifetime. Even better news is that living cells continually make new connections that replace at least some of the ones lost.

Still, the changes that occur do affect your cognitive processes to some degree. What do these changes mean for you?

For most people, it means that you may become a little more forgetful as you age — these are often momentary lapses of memory caused by inattention or distraction. Forgetfulness is normal in older adults, and it doesn't mean they have a dementia such as Alzheimer's disease. Other memory changes may become more common with age. These include:

Difficulty recalling names and facts. You may find it harder to remember information that you feel you should know, such as the date of your best friend's birthday or the title of a recent book you read. This can be frustrating at times when you need to remember information "on the spot." This explains why you may not be able to remember the name of the neighbor you run into at the grocery store until you're walking back out to your car!

Absentmindedness. Absentmindedness is often the culprit when you can't find your wallet or you overlook an appointment. It happens when you're so preoccupied with one thought that you tend to overlook everything else. It also can result from doing too many things at one time and not paying attention to any one thing.

Weakened memories. Memories that you don't often call upon will fade with time. Conversely, the memories that you recall regularly remain sharp. For many, this is common sense: You remember the things you think about most often.

Memory blocks. Have you been in a situation where you know what you want to say but you just can't think of the words to express it? Memory blocks may be the culprit when you find yourself saying, "The answer's right on the tip of my tongue!" This lapse often occurs because another persistent memory is blocking the concept you're looking for.

In addition to memory difficulties, other cognitive functions are vulnerable to aging. Your brain may require more processing and response time to complex problems compared to your 30- and 40-something counterparts. This may become evident with challenging visual input and complex construction tasks. When given the time to properly process this information, however, older adults often deliver solutions as accurately as those of young adults. So if you're someone who's always enjoyed jigsaw puzzles, you should be able to continue doing them well into old age — though you may find that the task takes a little longer to complete.

Making sense of new information can be more difficult as you age, as well. Even the healthiest people may notice a decline in their ability to learn new things beginning at about age 50. Let's say you've waited to learn to drive a car until old age. While the instructions given in a driver's education class may "click" right away for the teenagers, you'll likely need a little more time — and maybe a bit more instruction to learn the skills. This doesn't mean that you lose intelligence or can't think for yourself. On the contrary, most people remain both alert and able as they age — with mental performance staying the same well into the 80s and beyond.

Indeed, there are many important cognitive functions that are hardly affected by the normal aging process. The ability to focus, concentrate and create aren't diminished by age. Being able to use a rich vocabulary and to say what you mean actually increase with each passing year. Perhaps most importantly, however, age brings wisdom — the ability to use and enlighten others with the insight and knowledge you've gained from a lifetime of experiences.

A little reassurance

Before you read further in this book, understand this: While the possibility exists that any older adult can contract Alzheimer's disease, *having the disease is not a normal part of aging*. After all, minor memory lapses happen to almost everyone — especially as a person gets older. But only 3 percent of people ages 65 to 74 actually have Alzheimer's disease.

The truth is that Alzheimer's involves more than memory loss. Take the example of Mary at the beginning of this chapter. Although misplacing a purse or having to search the parking lot for a parked car may be frustrating and embarrassing, it doesn't mean she has Alzheimer's. For John, the struggle to find words could mean the age-related slowing down of mental processing and not the beginnings of dementia.

The very fact that both Mary and John are aware of forgetting things suggests that they probably don't have Alzheimer's. This is in contrast to the example of Hank, recounted in Chapter 1. Hank may sense things aren't quite right in his life, but he probably has trouble identifying exactly what those problems are.

If a family member or friend is exhibiting some of the signs of abnormal aging described in Chapter 1, don't assume that he or she has dementia. Appearances can be deceiving — just because you believe it looks like dementia and sounds like dementia doesn't make it dementia. You need a specialist's careful interpretation of the signs and symptoms.

Sometimes, when older adults feel especially lonely, worried or bored, they exhibit some of the symptoms associated with dementia. For example, coping with the death of a spouse can cause depression, confusion and emotional problems that may be mistaken for dementia. Instead of jumping to conclusions, become more informed (reading this book is a good start), and talk with a doctor you trust. The diagnosing of dementia is described in Chapter 3.

Diagnosing dementia

S arah is a 68-year-old widow who hasn't felt her normal self in weeks. In addition to her increasing forgetfulness, Sara is often confused and moody. She needs help doing simple chores around the house, and she finds herself snapping at neighbors and friends — something she never used to do. Her daughter is urging her to see a doctor, but Sarah's reluctant. She argues that if the family is willing to wait just a little longer, she'll work it out and "shake" the symptoms on her own. If she were being honest, however, Sarah might admit that she's afraid of going in for tests.

Like many people, Sarah hopes that what she doesn't know won't hurt her. But her daughter assures her that seeing a doctor is the right thing to do. The truth is that whatever the doctor finds out may make living much easier and help ease everyone's concerns. The sooner Sarah makes that appointment, the better the chances for some improvement in her life.

The importance of early diagnosis

It's estimated that more than 50 percent of people who have dementia never receive a diagnosis. Many, perhaps, don't realize they have a serious problem. They simply think that they're just "getting old." Or they may be concerned about the forgetfulness, the confusion and the mood swings they're experiencing but view them as separate problems and don't draw connections between them. Some may sense that they have a problem but don't *want* to receive a diagnosis. Like Sarah, they're afraid of the possibilities, including something serious like dementia.

It's true that if you're experiencing memory loss or abrupt mood changes, your doctor will likely consider dementia as a potential cause. But keep in mind that dementia is not the only possible cause of these symptoms. The earlier you make that appointment, undergo the evaluation and receive a diagnosis, the more options you're likely to have that may improve your symptoms and better your life — whether you have dementia or not.

It's estimated that 5 percent to 10 percent of people who have memory loss, confusion and other signs of dementia have a potentially reversible illness, such as metabolic problems, depression, drug interactions or thyroid problems. An earlier diagnosis generally makes treatment of these conditions easier.

In Sarah's case, for instance, doctors may find that her problems with memory and doing household chores — despite the annoyance they cause — are age-related and normal. What about her confusion and moodiness? Those could be a result of drug interactions from several new medications her doctor prescribed last month. By changing her prescriptions, Sarah could feel her life rapidly returning to normal.

On the other hand, doctors may perform a series of tests that make dementia the only possible cause. Though such a diagnosis may be difficult to hear, there are advantages to receiving the news early. Those affected can use this time to establish a support system, organize affairs and arrange for care in the days ahead. The earlier a person is diagnosed, the better the family can:

Prepare mentally and emotionally for the changes ahead. More time allows you to learn more about the disease, which can lessen anxiety and fear. It also allows family members to plan adequately for new living arrangements and day-to-day care.

Explore the treatment options. Although no drug exists that can stop or reverse the disorder, drugs do exist that may help treat the early-stage symptoms of dementia, such as Alzheimer's, and improve quality of life. Whether these drugs might possibly slow the progress of the disease is being studied.

Treat coexisting conditions. Many people with dementia also experience depression, anxiety or any one of several sleep disorders. Often, treating these conditions results in improved general health and potentially improved cognition.

Make important decisions regarding medical, legal and financial care. An early diagnosis may allow those affected with the disorder to actively participate with the family in important decisions that have to be made, particularly decisions that relate to care in later stages of the disease.

Solving the puzzle

While there are no definitive tests to determine that someone has dementia, doctors can be quite accurate in making the diagnosis. How do they do this?

A doctor starts by interviewing the person, as well as a family member or friend, to see if there has been a functional decline in the performance of daily activities. If there is a loss of function, the doctor will try to determine if this loss has been caused by a change in cognition. Following more examination, if the clinician feels that the functional decline is due to a loss of memory or concentration skills, for example, it's likely that dementia is present.

Next, the doctor must determine the cause of dementia. For help, the doctor may order procedures such as brain scans or blood tests. Based on these results, the doctor may conclude that a degenerative process such as Alzheimer's disease or a vascular process such as vascular cognitive impairment causes the dementia.

Using this method, doctors are able to make an accurate diagnosis of dementia about 90 percent of the time — which means there's a chance that the diagnosis may change if the signs and symptoms change. A diagnosis with 100 percent certainty can be accomplished with an autopsy, when the brain tissue can be removed and examined directly.

Criteria for a diagnosis

It's fair to say that dementia is a common condition among older adults — affecting as many as 10 percent of people older than age 65, and 25 percent to 47 percent of those older than age 85.

The official criteria most often used to diagnose dementia are established by the American Psychiatric Association and described in a handbook called the *Diagnostic and Statistical Manual of Mental Disorders*, fourth edition (referred to as DSM-IV).

Typically, the following criteria must be met in order for a physician to diagnose dementia:

1. The individual has multiple problems with different cognitive functions, which include the following:

    A. There must be memory problems, involving both recent and remote memory

       and

    B. There is one or more of the following:
      - Deterioration of language use or comprehension (aphasia)
      - Inability to carry out basic motor activities (apraxia)
      - Failure to recognize or identify objects (agnosia)
      - Disturbance of executive function — inability to make decisions and to think abstractly

2. The impairment of memory and other cognitive functions is so severe as to interfere with daily activities and personal relationships. These changes represent a significant decline from previous levels of functioning.

3. These changes don't occur exclusively during a period of delirium — a state of mental confusion, disordered speech and clouded consciousness sometimes mistaken for dementia.

The doctor may look for evidence of behavior change, such as depression, anxiety, irritability, and inappropriate actions or language. Although these aren't considered cognitive decline, they're common indicators of dementia — and often some of the earliest signs noticed by loved ones that something may be wrong.

A lack of insight — of understanding what's happening — may be common in the early stages. Those affected by dementia may not be aware of their memory loss or other cognitive deficits. They may make plans and express intentions that are not suitable for their current situations. A man in the early stages of dementia, for example, may insist on investing a lot of money into a new business in which he has never shown previous interest or aptitude. A woman with serious problems with vision and balance may announce that she's going on a vigorous hike.

Those affected by dementia may not observe accepted mores and social conventions. They may tell inappropriate jokes and disregard social niceties, such as being polite and keeping one's voice down. They may act overly friendly with complete strangers. And they may neglect basic personal hygiene, such as bathing, brushing teeth and wearing clean clothes.

Some may experience delusions and hallucinations. Delusions are false beliefs, which cause mistrust, suspicion and paranoia. Hallucinations involve seeing or hearing something that's not really there. For instance, it's not uncommon for a person with dementia to be convinced that there are unwelcome visitors in the home, although no one else sees these intruders.

Anxiety and agitation are symptoms that can make caring for a loved one with dementia especially difficult. Some people become physically and verbally aggressive, while others channel their agitation by continuously pacing or wandering away.

The signs and symptoms described above may be caused by conditions other than dementia. For that reason, it's important not to jump to dire conclusions if you or a loved one experiences them, especially if just one of these symptoms appears. Remember that dementia is a syndrome, or a collection of symptoms.

It's also vital not to self-diagnose, either by checking a symptoms list or taking a dementia "screening test," which can be found online or at the drugstore. Not only are such tests inaccurate, but also they may cause undue worry or a false sense of security if the results are misinterpreted. It bears repeating that no single test can unequivocally determine that you have dementia.

It's more important that you work with your doctor and other specialists recommended to you. They have the education, experience and resources needed to accurately assess all your symptoms, make a diagnosis and offer appropriate treatment plans.

Types of cognitive and functional decline

Dementia is defined by various forms of cognitive decline that have confusing and often similar sounding names, for example, aphasia, agnosia and apraxia. Here are easy-to-understand explanations of these common components of dementia.

Memory loss

Sometimes known as amnesia — though this term is somewhat outdated now— memory loss is the one symptom that's essential for a diagnosis of dementia. This common form of cognitive decline is marked by an inability to recall past events, either partially or in full. Problems with recent memory are often the earliest and most noticeable signs of this decline.

Language decline

Aphasia is the deterioration of an individual's ability to use and understand language. For example, those affected may have trouble coming up with the names of familiar people, places and objects. Their speech is often nonsensical, repetitive, and peppered with nonspecific words such as *thing* and *it*. They may have difficulty understanding spoken and written language.

Visuospatial decline

The word *visuospatial* is a result of combining the root words *visual* and *spatial*. It logically follows that people with visuospatial decline become disoriented easily and have difficulty with spatial tasks, for example, judging the height of a step or the distance around an obstacle. A person may have trouble finding a way to the bathroom in a house where he or she has lived for 30 years.

Decline of executive functioning

Executive functioning refers to decision making and the ability to carry out those decisions. People with an impairment of executive functioning will have trouble with abstract thoughts, so they tend to avoid situations that may require processing new information. Managing finances, outlining a report, organizing a family vacation or throwing a large party would prove too difficult for people with this form of cognitive decline.

Inability to recognize familiar objects

Agnosia describes the failure to recognize or identify objects despite being able to see, hear and feel them normally. For example, a person walks into a classroom and is not able to recognize the chairs and desks in that room. Or the person cannot identify the shapes of different eating utensils at the table. As dementia progresses, those affected with agnosia may have difficulty recognizing their children or spouses — or even their own reflections in the mirror.

Decline of motor activities

Apraxia is a problem with your ability to carry out motor activities — even though you're aware and your senses and motor skills are in working order. For instance, someone with apraxia may be unable to wave to a neighbor, although he or she sees the neighbor waving in greeting and understands what is expected in response. Apraxia may make daily activities such as feeding and dressing yourself almost impossible.

Attention deficit

People experiencing this form of cognitive decline will find it difficult to concentrate on words being spoken to them or on tasks they're attempting to accomplish. They feel scatterbrained and highly distractible, and able to focus on one thing for only brief periods of time.

Loss of muscle coordination

Ataxia is a lack of coordination while performing voluntary movements — those movements that you make a conscious decision to perform. People with ataxia may appear clumsy or unstable while walking or climbing stairs because their movements are often jerky and disjointed.

Common diagnostic procedures

Although a doctor may be your primary contact during the evaluation, a whole team of medical professionals may be involved in a diagnosis, including specialists such as a neurologist and psychiatrist. The basic evaluation includes a medical history, a physical examination, a neurological evaluation, and cognitive and neuropsychological tests. Some of these tests are used to assess the person's current levels of cognitive skill and the presence of altered brain function. Other tests are used to identify or eliminate other medical conditions as a cause of the symptoms. These tests also may help determine the specific type of dementia, if that's what the symptoms are pointing to.

Sometimes, the doctors may find that the dementia-like symptoms are actually caused by a treatable condition such as depression, medication use or a metabolic disorder. Other times, the doctors will conclude that the symptoms can only be dementia. They will use the test results to find ways to help ease the symptoms or improve the person's general quality of life.

The tests that you can expect during the diagnostic process include the following:

Medical history
Compiling a medical history generally starts the diagnostic process. To compile the history, the doctor will want to interview the person showing the symptoms, as well as someone he or she spends a lot of time with. Interviewing a spouse, family member or friend is important because it's often difficult to be objective and remember every detail when you're the one being interviewed. Plus, it allows the doctor to get another perspective on what are often subjective accounts involving feelings and behaviors.

The purpose of the interview is to identify any signs and symptoms associated with dementia and to create a chronology of events. The doctor will want to record personality and mood changes, and to assess how the person performs tasks now in comparison with his or her previous level of competence — including household chores, mental computations and social interactions.

Questions may include:
- What's your daily routine like?
- When were the first symptoms noticed?
- Have the symptoms gotten worse or have they remained relatively constant?
- Are the symptoms severe enough that they're beginning to interfere with daily activities?

The doctor may also ask questions about past or ongoing medical concerns, any over-the-counter or prescription medications being taken, a family history of dementia and other diseases, and the social and cultural background of the family.

Physical examination
Assessing the current status of a person's health is another critical step in the diagnostic process. Any number of physical factors, such as congestive heart failure, hypothyroidism, or vision and hearing

Preparing for an appointment
A medical history is an integral part of the diagnostic process. It's a good idea to prepare for the evaluation by jotting down the following information before the doctor appointment:
- Concern that made you seek an evaluation in the first place
- Changes you've noticed in your daily routine or how you go about performing common tasks
- Symptoms that you feel have become particular problems, including when they began, how frequently they recur and how they affect daily activities, such as driving, cooking or getting to scheduled appointments
- General outlook on life
- Current and past medical problems, including when they were diagnosed and what treatments were prescribed
- Family history of medical problems, including relationships and age when the problems were diagnosed
- Medications currently being taken, including both prescription and nonprescription medications — and don't forget herbal and dietary supplements

problems, may affect cognitive functions. This part of the diagnostic process may include:

- **General physical.** Identifies medical conditions that may be contributing to cognitive impairment or other symptoms
- **Electrocardiogram.** Records the heart's electric impulses as it pumps blood
- **Chest X-ray.** Measures cardiovascular health and checks for factors that may influence vascular cognitive impairment
- **Nutritional assessment.** Checks nutrition and weight status

Neurological evaluation

This series of tests focuses on physiological aspects of the brain and nervous system. Your doctor may test balance, sensation and other functions. A neurological exam may identify signs of Parkinson's disease, strokes, tumors or other medical conditions that can impair memory and cognition as well as physical function.

Mental status evaluation

To help determine which cognitive functions are affected, a clinician will assess the person's mental status. This assessment may include interviews and written tests to evaluate:

- Recent memory
- Remote memory
- Attention span
- Awareness of time and place
- Word comprehension, reading and writing
- Ability to perform daily activities

Additional evaluations may include doing simple calculations, language exercises (such as spelling a word backward) and drawing a simple design.

Neuropsychological tests

Neuropsychological tests are a more thorough type of cognitive testing that helps determine the nature and severity of impairment. The tests are designed to evaluate memory, language competency, and the ability to reason and problem solve. They also can assess the degree of coordination between a person's vision and muscular movement. Test results can help indicate the person's ability to handle a variety of common but complex tasks, such as driving a car and managing finances. They also may help in the decision of whether it's safe for someone to live alone, or to what degree he or she should have assistance at home.

Common neuropsychological tests

To test ...	The doctor might ask the person ...
Recent memory	To learn a list of words and repeat them, then recall them after a delay of several minutes, and then identify them from a longer list of words
Remote memory	To relate personal history — such as childhood recollections, where the person went to school, when he or she got married, or the town where the person lived when the children were young
Language skills	To name common objects in the room, such as a desk, light switch or curtain; to follow commands, such as repeating a simple phrase or pointing at different items in succession
Motor skills	To stack blocks, arrange pencils in a specific design or demonstrate how he or she brushes teeth
Executive functions	To count to 10, point out the similarities and differences in related words, or list words that begin with a certain letter

These tests may be critical for differentiating between dementia and a concurrent condition such as depression, especially in the early stages of dementia. They may also help in distinguishing between different types of dementia that have common signs and symptoms, such as Alzheimer's disease, dementia with Lewy bodies and frontotemporal dementia.

Possible diagnostic procedures

If a doctor has conducted the diagnostic tests listed above but is still looking for answers, he or she may recommend other procedures. These tests may eliminate a potential, nondementia cause or reveal more about a particular symptom.

Laboratory blood tests and urine tests can help pinpoint a treatable cause for the symptoms, such as thyroid problems, anemia, infections, medication and vitamin levels, and other factors. For example, a routine blood test can measure vitamin B levels as well as liver and thyroid functions. A urine test may detect the presence of certain drugs or uncover a urinary tract infection, which can cause confusion or declining cognition in some older adults.

A psychiatric assessment may be recommended as well. This helps determine if the person has depression or another condition that may mimic dementia. This assessment may reveal certain cognitive patterns that are clues to the underlying condition.

A doctor may also recommend a brain scan, using sophisticated, noninvasive technology, to get a clear picture of what's going on inside your brain. Brain imaging can't replace standard diagnostic procedures, but it may provide a clue or confirm a suspicion that helps identify the cause of the symptoms.

There are two different types of brain imaging that the medical team might recommend to help with the diagnosis: structural imaging and functional imaging.

Structural imaging
Structural imaging provides pictures of the shape and volume of internal structures of your brain, and may be used to help detect strokes, tumors, brain injury, hydrocephalus or other structural

abnormalities. The procedure can also reveal whether there's atrophy (shrinkage) of the brain. You may have already heard of the two types of structural imaging:

Computerized tomography. Computerized tomography (CT scan) is an imaging technique that's used extensively in diagnostic evaluations of the brain and other organs. As you lie on a table, the CT scanner rotates around you, emitting a series of thin X-ray beams that pass through you at different angles. A computer processes these scans and combines them into 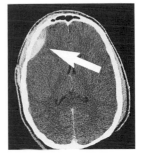 a single, detailed, cross-sectional image. A CT scan makes organs that are difficult or impossible to see on an ordinary X-ray more visible and visible in greater detail. The example of a CT scan above reveals the buildup of blood in the brain caused by a ruptured artery (see arrow).

Magnetic resonance imaging. Rather than using X-rays to produce an image, magnetic resonance imaging (MRI) uses magnetic fields and radio waves. The machine detects energy signals emitted by the atoms that make up body tissues and constructs images based on that 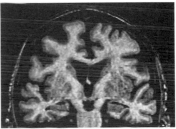 information. The images produced with this technology are more detailed and may show slightly different tissues than those of a CT scan. Magnetic resonance images, such as the example shown here, are particularly useful for evaluating areas of the brain because of the detail they reveal about white and gray matter.

Functional imaging

Functional imaging creates pictures of brain activity rather than of brain structures. It does so by detecting changes in chemical composition or blood flow in the tissues. The images can help clarify relationships between specific mental functions — for example, listening to a conversation or recalling a memory — and activity taking place in different regions of the brain — for example, in the temporal lobe or limbic system. Using this procedure, a doctor may be able to observe activity in a part of the brain that suggests Alzheimer's disease rather than frontotemporal dementia, for example.

Types of functional imaging include:

Positron emission tomography (PET). Positron emission tomography is an imaging technique that detects emissions from a small amount of radioactive material that's injected into the body. Two different detectors placed on opposite sides of the body record the emissions. This technique has the advantage of being able to reveal the way in which various tissues actually use energy.

Single-photon emission computed tomography (SPECT). Similar to a PET scan, a small amount of radioactive material is injected into the body. A camera that can detect the radioactive material rotates around the head to create three-dimensional images of blood flow and brain activity.

Functional magnetic resonance imaging (fMRI). Similar to an MRI, an fMRI uses magnetism — in this case, the magnetic properties of blood — to reveal activity in different areas of the brain and to detect changes in this activity over short periods of time. The fMRI technology is used primarily for research and generally is not involved in the diagnostic process.

Diagnosing a type of dementia

The various tests and procedures described in this chapter may help a doctor reach a diagnosis of dementia. But that's not the end of the examination. The doctor must now consider an even more complex question: What kind of dementia is it?

As stated previously, many conditions — from vitamin deficiencies to Alzheimer's disease — can cause the signs and symptoms associated with dementia. And although the different types of dementia have symptoms in common, each type develops in a characteristic pattern with variations that are often subtle. For example, both Alzheimer's disease and frontotemporal dementia (FTD) involve memory loss as a primary symptom. But in Alzheimer's, memory impairment is often one of the first symptoms that's noticed. In FTD, emotional problems often develop first, with memory loss occurring at a later stage of the disease.

So how do doctors go about trying to identify what kind of dementia a person has? The same way that they diagnose dementia in the first place — through a systematic process of evaluation, testing, analysis and comparison.

Once again, doctors must consider the various signs and symptoms collectively in order to narrow the field of potential causes. If the person hasn't exhibited any emotional problems and a brain scan shows no damage to the frontal or temporal lobes, for instance, frontotemporal dementia isn't likely to be the culprit and can be moved down the list of possible causes.

Sometimes determining a type of dementia is easier than at other times. For example, if a person's medical history shows a history of strokes and the person started to experience cognitive decline shortly after the strokes, doctors will take that as a good indication of vascular cognitive impairment.

Other times, however, additional testing and lab work may be required to determine the cause of dementia. Memory loss and cognitive decline may clearly suggest dementia in someone, for instance, but it may not be until Parkinson's, HIV, brain tumors and myriad other causes have been ruled out — and crucial brain scans have been studied — that the doctor may diagnose the cause as Alzheimer's disease.

Sometimes, even after completion of all the tests, the type of dementia still cannot be determined. For example, several characteristic symptoms of dementia with Lewy bodies are the same as those of Alzheimer's disease. The same may be said for the cognitive symptoms of vascular cognitive impairment and Alzheimer's. To add to the challenge, these different forms of dementia can co-exist, with a single person being affected by more than one type of dementia. It's possible for someone to have Alzheimer's disease and dementia with Lewy bodies or vascular cognitive impairment at the same time.

Even if doctors are unable to determine the exact type of dementia that a person has, that doesn't change the level of care that a person will receive. He or she can still be made comfortable, can still plan for the future and, when appropriate, can still receive treatment for his or her symptoms.

Using brain imaging

Although brain imaging — such as a CT scan, magnetic resonance image (MRI) or PET scan — can't diagnose dementia, it can be helpful in differentiating among the different types of dementia. If dementia has been diagnosed, doctors may use the images to look for specific changes in the brain that indicate, for instance, whether a person has Alzheimer's disease or vascular dementia. The three examples below show how brain imaging helps doctors diagnose different types of dementia.

Alzheimer's disease

Brain images from people with Alzheimer's often show noticeable atrophy (shrinkage) of brain structures associated with memory, such as the hippocampus. The magnetic resonance images below compare the brain of a person without dementia (left) with that of a person in the moderate stage of Alzheimer's disease (right). The progression of Alzheimer's is indicated on the right by a hippocampus that's noticeably shrunken (circled in white) and interior cavities of the brain that have enlarged and filled with cerebrospinal fluid (indicated by the arrow).

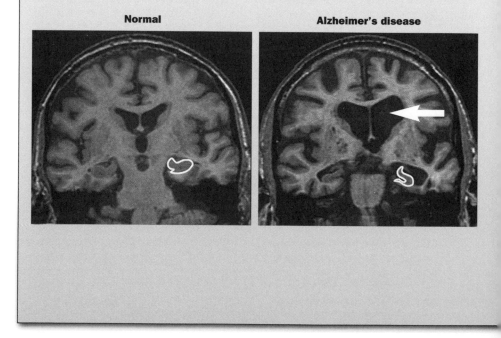

Normal   Alzheimer's disease

Frontotemporal dementia
In FTD, a magnetic resonance image or CT scan can reveal shrinkage (atrophy) in the frontal and temporal lobes of the brain (indicated by the arrow). In the early stages of FTD, when atrophy may not be prominent, functional imaging tests such as a PET or SPECT

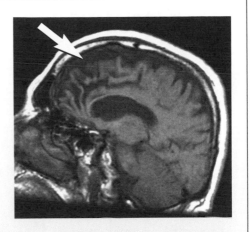

scan may show decreased metabolism in these lobes.

Note that while Alzheimer's disease and FTD will both show evidence of brain atrophy, the areas where the shrinkage takes place are typically different — helping to differentiate one type of dementia from the other.

Vascular cognitive impairment
When testing for vascular cognitive impairment, doctors look to CT scans or magnetic resonance images for signs of stroke. Brain scans for someone with vascular cognitive impairment typically show lesions and other damaged areas caused by either multiple small strokes

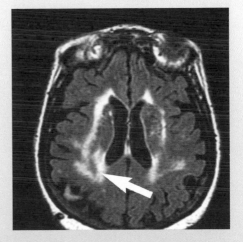

or a single stroke. In this image, damage to brain tissue caused by stroke appears as distinct areas of white (see arrow) in the interior of the brain.

What happens after diagnosis?

Being diagnosed with dementia is a frightening experience. You'll need to give yourself time to work through a variety of feelings and to adjust emotionally.

Don't be afraid to ask family and friends for help. A doctor, nurse or psychologist can work with you and your family to develop strategies to manage symptoms of the disease as it progresses. He or she can help you determine the right time and the manner in which to tell others of the diagnosis. There also may be resources in your community that can provide valuable advice and assistance, such as a local chapter of Area Agencies on Aging or the Alzheimer's Association.

If you've been diagnosed with a specific type of dementia, take advantage of this time to learn more about it. Many types of dementia, including Alzheimer's, frontotemporal dementia, dementia with Lewy bodies, vascular cognitive impairment and more, are explored in depth in later chapters.

If a loved one has received a diagnosis of Alzheimer's disease and you want to learn more about the disease, this is also the book for you. Becoming familiar with the type of dementia affecting your loved one will help you anticipate changes and prepare for the experiences ahead. More about learning how to cope with a diagnosis of dementia can be found in the Action Guide for Caregivers, located at the back of this book.

T his section is intended to help you better understand Alzheimer's disease by seeing what happens to the normal brain as the disease develops and progresses.

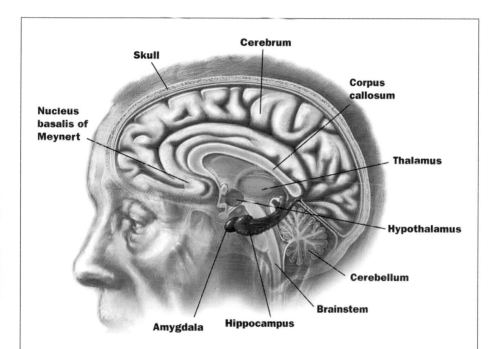

Internal structures of the brain

The brain is composed of three main regions:

Cerebrum. The cerebrum, which makes up the bulk of the brain, processes information from the outside world, controls voluntary movement, and regulates conscious thought and mental activity. Several essential parts of the brain, such as the hippocampus, amygdala, thalamus and hypothalamus, lie deep inside the cerebrum.

Cerebellum. The much smaller cerebellum controls balance and coordination.

Brainstem. The brainstem relays information between the brain and spinal cord and controls automatic functions that keep us alive — heart rate, blood pressure and breathing.

The onset and progression of Alzheimer's disease

Alzheimer's disease attacks the brain by destroying its most basic component, the nerve cell (neuron), which facilitates cell communication. Neuron loss occurs first in the hippocampus and spreads to the amygdala (purple shading). In its moderate stage, the disease spreads farther, into the cerebral cortex. In the severe stage, most of the brain is damaged, except for the occipital lobe, at the back of the brain.

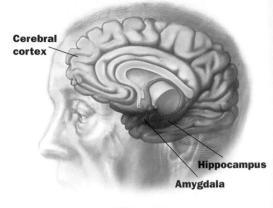

Cerebral cortex

Hippocampus

Amygdala

Sagittal section

Mild stage

Changes in brain structure and activity

This series of magnetic resonance imaging (MRI) scans shows how the brain's hippocampus (circled in red) shrinks as the disease worsens. The hippocampus is critical to memory storage and recall. This explains why memory loss is often one of the first signs of Alzheimer's disease.

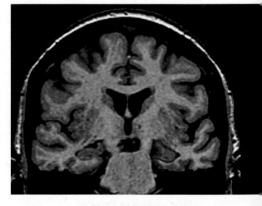

Coronal section

Normal brain

This series of positron emission tomography (PET) scans shows a reduction in brain activity as Alzheimer's disease progresses. The red, orange and white colors indicate areas of intense activity, with white being the most intense. Cool colors, such as blue and green, represent low activity. As you can see, the white areas are reduced dramatically as the disease progresses. Reduced brain activity leads to a decline in mental and physical abilities.

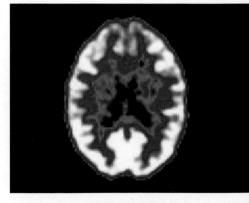

Axial section

Normal brain

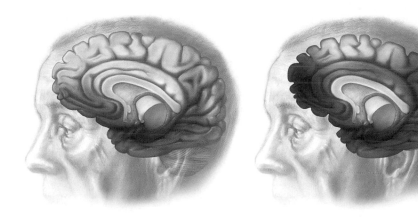

Moderate stage   Severe stage

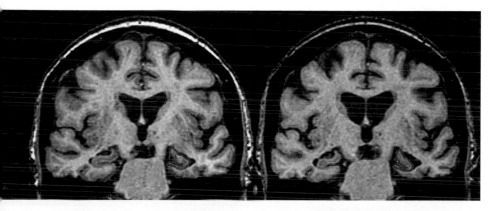

Mild cognitive impairment   **Alzheimer's disease**

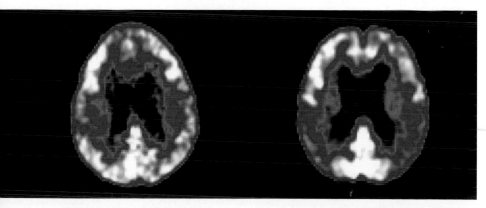

Mild cognitive impairment   **Alzheimer's disease**

Formation of plaques

Dense deposits of protein and cellular material outside and around neurons, called plaques, are one of the hallmarks of Alzheimer's disease. Plaques are formed from a substance called amyloid precursor protein (APP). In Alzheimer's disease, something causes the APP molecule to be snipped at a different location than normal, making the fragment longer, "stickier" and less able to dissolve. The insoluble fragments clump together and form into plaques.

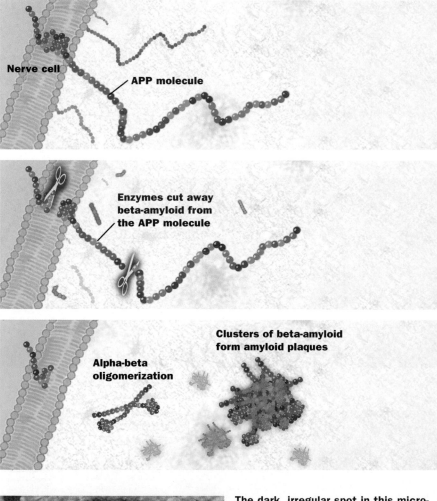

Nerve cell

APP molecule

Enzymes cut away beta-amyloid from the APP molecule

Clusters of beta-amyloid form amyloid plaques

Alpha-beta oligomerization

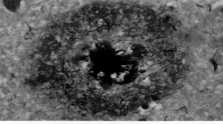

The dark, irregular spot in this micro-photograph is a dense core of an amyloid plaque. The discoloration surrounding the core indicates inflammation.

Formation of tangles

Nerve cells (neurons) have an internal support structure, which includes components called microtubules. A protein known as tau helps stabilize the microtubules. In Alzheimer's disease, the chemical makeup of tau changes, causing the tau to unravel and destabilize the microtubules. The disintegrating pieces of tau clump together within the cell to form tangles.

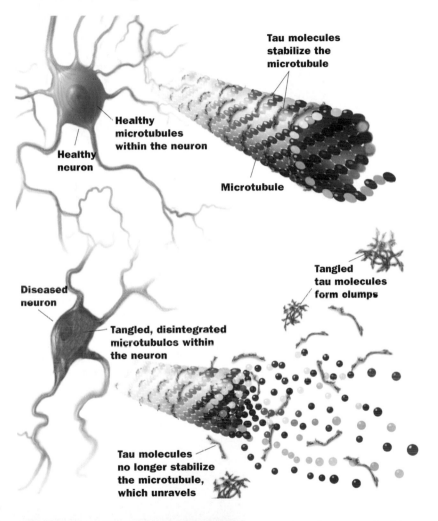

Tau molecules stabilize the microtubule

Healthy microtubules within the neuron

Healthy neuron

Microtubule

Tangled tau molecules form clumps

Diseased neuron

Tangled, disintegrated microtubules within the neuron

Tau molecules no longer stabilize the microtubule, which unravels

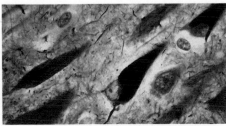

The dark, solid masses in this microphotograph are the collapsed structures of neurons.

Shrinkage of the brain

This series of illustrations shows how the brain gradually becomes smaller in size as Alzheimer's disease progresses. Note the widening creases in the cerebral cortex. Also note how the brain's cavities (ventricles) enlarge.

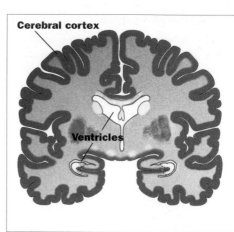

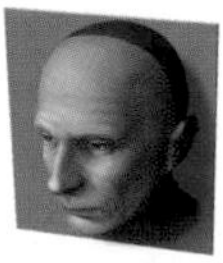

Normal brain

Coronal section

Shown here are three MRI scans of a woman who was 77 years old when the first image was taken. Note the shrinkage of the brain and the increasing size of the central ventricle (see arrows).

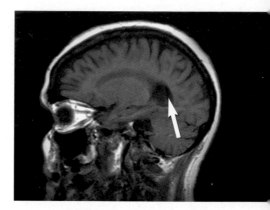

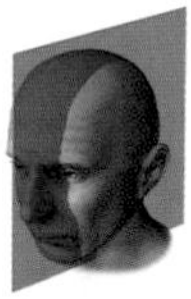

Normal brain, 1994

Sagittal section

Other dementias

Frontotemporal dementia (FTD) is the name for a diverse group of neurodegenerative disorders that primarily affect the frontal and temporal lobes of the brain. Note the difference in the front part of the brain in these images showing a normal brain and one damaged by FTD (side and front views).

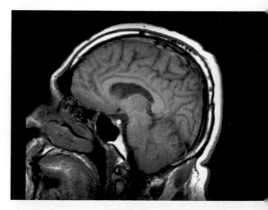

Normal

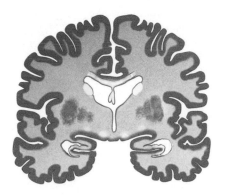
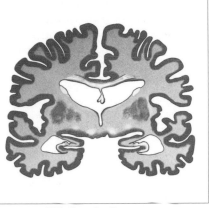

Mild cognitive impairment   **Alzheimer's disease**

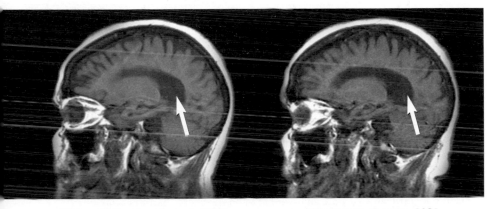

Mild cognitive impairment, 1997   **Alzheimer's disease, 2001**

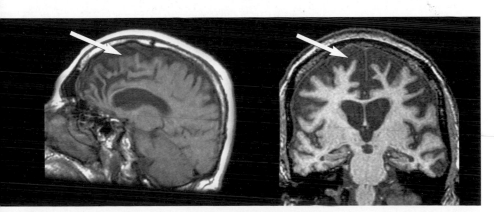

Frontotemporal dementia

Vascular cognitive impairment results when blood flow to the brain is interrupted, most often due to a stroke, causing cell death in specific areas. The damaged areas (infarcts) can result in memory loss and changes in reasoning and emotions. The white areas in these images indicate loss of blood supply. The image on the left shows a large area of brain damage, while the image on the right shows several small areas of brain damage.

Axial section

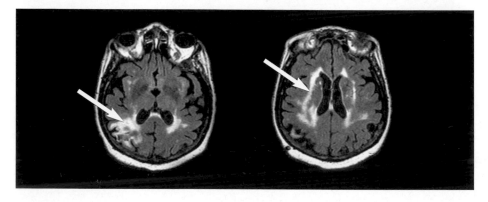

Research trends

Scientists are hoping to find a substance in the body (biological marker) that could help identify people at high risk of dementia, enabling these individuals to receive treatment before the onset of symptoms. One technique being studied is a type of tracer called Pittsburgh Compound B (PIB), which sticks to amyloid plaques in the brain. The tracer can be seen on PET scans. An example is shown here. Note the difference between the normal (control) brain and the brain affected by Alzheimer's disease. The bright colors (yellow and orange) indicate where the tracer has been retained, indicating amyloid plaques. The presence of brain plaques doesn't mean that an individual has Alzheimer's disease, but it becomes a cause of active investigation.

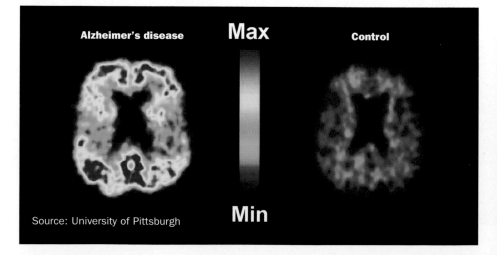

Alzheimer's disease

Max

Control

Min

Source: University of Pittsburgh

Part 2

Alzheimer's disease

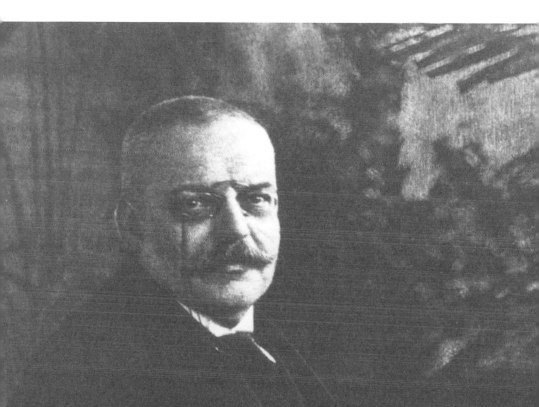

The year 2007 is the 100th anniversary of Dr. Alois Alzheimer's published account of the disease that now bears his name. The following chapters describe how much progress has been made in fighting this terrible disorder.

Chapter 4

The basics of Alzheimer's disease

Alzheimer's disease is the most common cause of dementia among adults in their 60s and older. It's a cruel and unrelenting illness that ravages the mind. Alzheimer's slowly robs a person of intellect and memory, impairs good judgment and destroys the ability to communicate and learn. The disease causes behavior change and extreme emotional swings. As the mind gradually deteriorates, the body loses its ability to function.

The course that Alzheimer's disease may take is highly variable from one person to the next. It may run anywhere from 2 to 20 years after the initial signs and symptoms appear. The disease is terminal, and death generally occurs from the complications of being immobile and unable to eat or drink — which include pneumonia and other infections, malnutrition, dehydration and problems with the circulatory system.

How Alzheimer's disease develops

Alzheimer's disease affects the brain by destroying its most basic components — neurons, or the nerve cells that relay information throughout the body. The disease also wreaks havoc with the synapses — communication points between the cells — further impairing the communication process. How and why neuron death occurs is still a subject of debate, although scientists are learning more about the possible causes (see Chapter 5 for more information on the potential causes of Alzheimer's).

One thing that scientists do have an accurate picture of is where the problems start. Neuron loss occurs first in the region of the hippocampus, part of the limbic system located in the central brain. The hippocampus acts as the central switchboard of your memory system. That's why memory loss is often associated with the early stages of Alzheimer's. There also may be disorientation and the loss of visuospatial function — the perception of where objects or places are located in relation to each other.

After the hippocampus, Alzheimer's disease attacks other parts of the limbic system, including the amygdala. And the disease spreads from there to the frontal, parietal and temporal lobes of the cerebral cortex. As neuron communication is damaged or destroyed in these areas, other cognitive capabilities are impaired, such as lan-

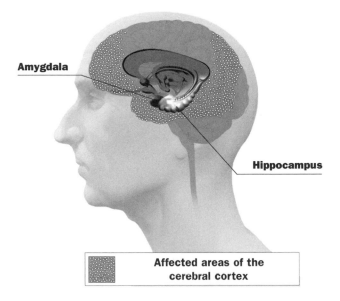

Amygdala

Hippocampus

Affected areas of the
cerebral cortex

The early stages of Alzheimer's disease

The hippocampus, a key component of the memory system, is generally affected at the onset of the disease. From there, the disease spreads to other parts of the limbic system and to the cerebral cortex.

guage skills and executive functions, including the abilities to plan and make decisions. Gradually, the disease robs people of their facility to perform simple tasks, routine self-care and household duties that they may have done for many years. Since the limbic system is the part of the brain that influences instincts and emotions, neuron loss in this area also may explain the aggressive behavior and paranoia often seen in people with Alzheimer's.

In addition, Alzheimer's disease causes a loss of nerve cells at a location deep within the brain called the basal nucleus of Meynert. This area is rich in a neurotransmitter called acetylcholine (uh-set-ul-KOE-leen), and damage to the nucleus causes a sharp drop in acetylcholine levels. Acetylcholine plays an important role in the formation and retrieval of memories, compounding the memory loss due to the disease's impact on the hippocampus.

Alzheimer's disease decreases the levels of other important neurotransmitters in the brain, such as dopamine, glutamate, norepinephrine and serotonin. The chart at the bottom of this page indicates what other brain functions may be impaired or lost when these neurotransmitters are at reduced levels.

Eventually, Alzheimer's spreads throughout the brain. As more and more nerve cells die, brain mass shrinks. A person with Alzheimer's ultimately loses some or all of his or her ability to communicate, recognize familiar faces and objects, control behavior and satisfy basic physical urges, such as the need to eat or to urinate. In the final stages of Alzheimer's disease, most people are bedridden and completely dependent on others for care.

Neurotransmitter levels affected by Alzheimer's

Neurotransmitter	Primary function
acetylcholine	attention, learning and memory
dopamine	physical movement
glutamate	learning and remote memory
norepinephrine	emotional response
serotonin	mood and anxiety

Stages of Alzheimer's disease

People who develop Alzheimer's will experience the disease in very different ways. This includes the rate at which the disease progresses and the type and severity of the symptoms. These differences depend on many factors, including age, personality, physical health, family history, and cultural and ethnic backgrounds.

Nevertheless, certain patterns are common in almost everyone with Alzheimer's over the course of the disease. Using these patterns as symptomatic benchmarks, medical professionals describe the development of Alzheimer's in stages ranging from mild to severe. Some experts divide this range into three stages, others into four or more. What distinguishes one stage from another is the new appearance of or a change in the various indicators, in terms of cognition (how a person thinks), behavior (how a person acts) and function (how a person is able to perform basic tasks).

In this book, three stages are used to categorize Alzheimer's disease: mild, moderate and severe. The description of each stage is for general purposes and may not fit a particular individual's circumstances exactly. Some of the signs and symptoms that are described may overlap from one stage to the next. Other signs and symptoms may never occur in some people.

Mild Alzheimer's

Increased forgetfulness is the most common complaint in the early stages of Alzheimer's disease. At first, the person may have difficulty with recent memory — new information such as names or appointments — even while remote memories remain intact. Usually, memory loss associated with Alzheimer's presents itself as a new and more intense pattern of forgetfulness that persists.

Still, the early signs of Alzheimer's are often hidden and subtle, making it difficult to recognize that something is actually wrong. There may be slight problems with communicating or uncharacteristic changes in personality. It may be easy for the person to become disoriented in his or her daily routine.

Even if people sense problems, they may not associate the changes with an illness. Many people in the early stages seem to be less aware and less concerned about their problems than are family and friends — this lack of awareness may itself be an early symptom of the disease. Some of the earliest signs and symptoms of Alzheimer's include:

- Not remembering recent events
- Asking the same questions repeatedly
- Getting lost in conversations and having problems finding the right word
- Not being able to complete familiar tasks, for example, someone who loves to cook having difficulties with a recipe
- Having problems with abstract thought, for example, uncertainty over using a credit card for financial transactions
- Misplacing items in inappropriate places, such as putting a watch, wallet or handbag in the refrigerator
- Undergoing sudden, intense changes in mood or behavior with no apparent reasons for the change
- Showing an inability to concentrate for more than a few minutes or to take initiative and complete projects
- Showing less interest in what's going on in the surroundings
- Showing an indifference toward personal appearance, for example, being unwashed, uncombed and poorly dressed
- Not observing normal courtesies to others, for example, ignoring greetings and simple questions
- Feeling disoriented about time and place, for example, uncertainty about the general locations of stores in town
- Becoming lost while driving on familiar streets

Even as the mild stage of Alzheimer's develops, the person may still be employed and trying to go about doing business as usual. Difficulties at work may be passed off as stress, lack of sleep, fatigue or simply a part of getting older. The person may try to compensate for memory problems by sticking to places and routines that are familiar and not entering into new or strange situations. The growing awareness of memory loss may lead to feelings of anger, frustration and helplessness. It's not unusual for a person to take these emotions out on others. Depression also is common at the mild stage. Depression is a serious condition that should be evaluated and treated as soon as possible.

What does it feel like to have Alzheimer's?

This was a question asked by members of Mayo Clinic's Alzheimer's Disease Research Center to a group of people who had received a diagnosis in the mild stage of Alzheimer's. How they responded was surprisingly revealing. While some interviewees were philosophical, others were more pragmatic.

"Loss of independence. It doesn't feel right to become more dependent on others by letting them get the idea that you can't do anything. I give in and let others take over completely. You lose out when you let others take over. We need to slow down so I can stay involved."

"Fear. You hear it's so debilitating and that gets you down."

"When they hear Alzheimer's, people back up like you've got a 'disease.' Almost like you should be ashamed. Like they are wondering if it's catchy or if maybe she's going to die soon."

"Expectations others have for me are often too high or too low. I can't keep up with my spouse. It's quicker and easier to let my spouse take over."

"I need to be reminded of tasks or activities."

"I don't recognize places when we go for drives. That scares me."

"It takes me much longer to remember why I went into a room."

"I need to work at a slower pace. People around me seem like they are on a merry-go-round — going faster and faster. I can't keep up. I want to stay active, but I need to take more time to do things."

Moderate Alzheimer's

At the moderate stage, the warning signs that before had seemed out-of-place occurrences have now become more obvious. The individual may not only be experiencing memory loss but also having difficulty thinking clearly and exercising good judgment. He or she likely needs help with many day-to-day activities, including personal care. Moods may change literally from moment to moment.

These developments alert family members or friends that something is definitely wrong. If there had been any reluctance to see a doctor before, these new concerns may prompt a doctor visit now. Signs and symptoms of the moderate stage include:

- Forgetting to turn off appliances such as the iron and stove.
- Consistently forgetting to take medications even with constant reminders and mnemonic devices.
- Having difficulty with tasks involving calculation and planning, such as balancing a checkbook, paying bills, going grocery shopping and planning dinner.
- Having difficulty with tasks that require skilled movements such as tying shoelaces and using utensils.
- Losing the ability to communicate and interact, including reading and writing.
- Exhibiting extreme behaviors, such as aggressiveness, withdrawal and outbursts of anger.
- Behaving inappropriately in public, for example, talking out loud and interrupting conversations.
- Feeling increasingly agitated and restless, particularly at night
- Sleeping for excessively long periods of time or hardly sleeping at all. Some people may sleep 10 to 12 hours at night and still nap during the day, while others may sleep only two to four hours at night.
- Having false beliefs (delusions) or seeing or hearing something that's not really there (hallucinations).

A diagnosis of Alzheimer's can be a trying time for anyone thrust into the unanticipated role of caregiver, whether it's a spouse, sibling or other family member or friend. It takes awhile to develop a new perspective on the relationship between caregiver and the person who has just received the diagnosis.

Where is my wife?

This haunting question was asked of a wife, caring for her husband with Alzheimer's disease. She describes the changes that occurred in their relationship in this way:

"It is heartbreaking for your spouse not to know you. But I have learned not to let it get to me. I tell my husband that his wife will soon be back or, if he persists, that she has gone to visit family.

At times, he tells me that his wife has gone to visit family, and I should sleep in the guest room. Well, I tell him that this bed is just like mine and I would sleep better in it. He will get in bed and sleep at the farthest edge. But before he goes to sleep, he reaches over and holds my hand and kisses me good night."

— Edna L.

Severe Alzheimer's

In the severe stage of Alzheimer's, the disease has progressed to a point where the person is no longer able to think or reason. Self-awareness seems to have disappeared completely. The essential tasks of living, such as bathing, dressing, eating and going to the bathroom, require a caregiver's full assistance. The person's personality may have changed completely. Motor activities have deteriorated to the point where he or she can no longer walk, sit up or communicate. In fact, the person seems unmotivated to move at all without prompts from others. Signs and symptoms at this severe stage of the disease include:

- Having little or no memory, be it recent or remote
- Having difficulty with speaking and understanding words
- Showing little or no emotion
- Grasping objects or people and not letting go
- Having difficulty recognizing others — perhaps not even recognizing himself or herself when looking in a mirror
- Needing assistance with all personal care, including using the toilet, bathing, dressing, eating and moving around
- Experiencing frequent incontinence due to lack of bladder and bowel control

- Feeling increasingly weak and sleeping more
- Being highly susceptible to infections
- Having difficulty chewing and swallowing, and because of these problems, losing weight

A person in the final stage of Alzheimer's has become bed-ridden. His or her body systems are severely weakened, which increases the risk of developing other health problems. Because of the weakened systems, the effect of these added health problems frequently is more severe for a person with Alzheimer's than for someone without the disease. As a result, the cause of death is rarely Alzheimer's itself, and more often a secondary infection such as pneumonia. Death occurs, on average, about six to eight years following recognition of the symptoms as dementia.

Sample case of Alzheimer's

A man brought his 67-year-old wife to the doctor because of serious concerns about memory loss. His wife was well educated and an entrepreneur who had owned her own business for many years. Now, increasingly, she was unable to remember appointments, easily confused her orders and needed constant help with finances. She could no longer go on business trips for fear of muddling her itinerary and forgetting purchases. Outside of work, she had withdrawn from social activities she long enjoyed. And recently, she left food cooking on the stove unattended, resulting in a small kitchen fire.

The woman had no serious medical problems, took no medications and passed an initial physical examination, which showed nothing significantly wrong. Mental status testing, however, revealed mild naming problems and disorientation to the exact date. Further testing indicated short-term memory impairment and problems with language and calculations. A diagnosis was made of Alzheimer's disease.

Criteria for a diagnosis

If a doctor, following an examination, is fairly certain that a person has Alzheimer's — short of a brain biopsy or autopsy (only these can provide a definitive diagnosis) — he or she will make a diagnosis of "probable" Alzheimer's. In order for such a diagnosis to be made, the following criteria are required:

- The dementia is confirmed by a clinical exam (see Chapter 3 for more on clinical testing for dementia).
- Problems occur in at least two areas of cognitive function, one of which must be memory. Other functions that may be affected include language, visuospatial perception, simple numerical calculation and planning or another intellectual skill.
- Problems in the areas of cognitive function are getting progressively worse.
- There's no delirium or a disturbance of consciousness.
- Onset of the symptoms occurs between ages 40 and 90 (usually after age 65).
- Any other possible causes for the dementia are absent.

If the doctor believes that Alzheimer's disease is the primary cause of the signs and symptoms but thinks that another dementing disorder is present and affecting the disease process, the diagnosis may be one of "possible" Alzheimer's. The likely presence of a second dementing disorder may affect treatment options because the diagnosis is less certain. These disorders are described on pages 78-79 and in greater detail in later chapters of this book.

Conditions that may accompany Alzheimer's

Certain conditions, other than the dementing disorders referred to above, may develop at the same time as Alzheimer's. The symptoms can obscure or complicate a diagnosis of Alzheimer's. They may also hasten or increase the severity of mental decline. The fact that many of these conditions are treatable emphasizes the importance of an early diagnosis. Conditions that commonly coexist with Alzheimer's include depression, anxiety and sleep disorders.

Depression

Among people with a diagnosis of Alzheimer's disease (AD), about 20 percent to 30 percent experience significant depression at some point during the course of the disease. It's especially common during the early stages of Alzheimer's when social isolation, diminishing mental and physical abilities, and a loss of independence often occur. Brief periods of discouragement and apathy may be natural in such circumstances, but prolonged despondency is not.

Although coexistence is common, scientists aren't sure of the exact relationship between depression and dementia. Studies indicate that chronic feelings of sadness or worthlessness among people with Alzheimer's may be linked to an awareness of mental decline — despite the fact that many people with Alzheimer's lose insight into their behavior and abilities early in the disease process. Other research has found that the biological changes caused by Alzheimer's may intensify genetic predisposition to depression. Some studies suggest that the symptoms of depression, such as apathy and lack of motivation, may be among the earliest signs of AD. Other studies point to the idea that the presence of depression may increase your chances of developing Alzheimer's.

What's clear is that depression has a strong effect on quality of life for the person with Alzheimer's and for his or her caregiver. In addition to the emotional problems, depression can lead to weight loss and physical frailty. For more signs and symptoms of depression, see pages 15-16. Depression is also associated with an earlier placement in nursing homes, greater disability involving daily living skills and physical aggression toward caregivers. In addition, depression in a person with Alzheimer's increases the chances of depression in caregivers.

Diagnosing depression in a person with Alzheimer's can be especially challenging. This is due, in part, to the person's growing inability to describe how he or she feels. Another complicating factor is that many adults have been socialized to think that it's OK to be physically sick but not OK to admit to feelings of sadness or loneliness. Experts encourage caregivers or anyone else involved in the daily life of the person to take part in doctor visits to provide a more complete picture of the person's moods.

Counseling and nondrug therapy can be helpful, especially for people with mild depression. A professional therapist can help a person with Alzheimer's to develop daily routines and find enjoyable activities, and help caregivers learn problem-solving and coping skills. Sometimes, making use of adult day services can provide a needed break for both the person with Alzheimer's and his or her caregiver. Also, antidepressants can help relieve more severe symptoms of depression, such as extreme apathy, refusal to eat or drink, and suicidal or violent thoughts.

Anxiety

Anxiety is a sense of fear about an impending event, about something that's going to happen in the near future. A moderate amount of anxiety can be good — it can motivate you or help you respond to danger. But persistent anxiety affecting your day-to-day life can develop into a full-fledged anxiety disorder.

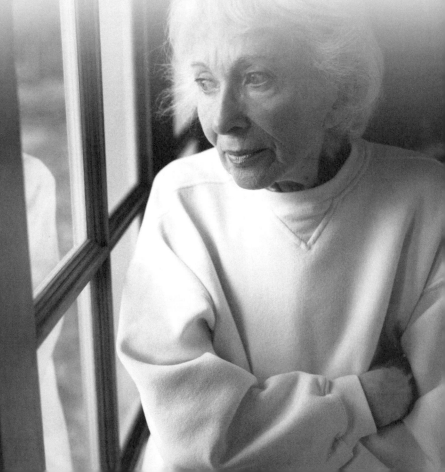

The symptoms of anxiety — fearfulness, agitation, apprehension, fidgeting or pacing, excessive worry, restlessness and even anger — are common among people with Alzheimer's. Research indicates that these symptoms occur in 80 percent or more of people with Alzheimer's disease. In addition, anxiety and depression often occur together.

Anxiety seems to be associated closely with many troublesome behaviors that may occur in someone with Alzheimer's. These include wandering, inappropriate sexual conduct, hallucinations, verbal threats and physical abuse. These behaviors are frequently reasons for placing someone in a nursing home. Treating anxiety effectively may improve the symptoms and, in turn, reduce the stress and fatigue that affect the caregiver.

Treatment for anxiety generally employs a strategy to manage the behavior. A common method for managing excess worry, irritability or restlessness is to identify the behavior that's causing concern, find out what may be causing it and adapt the person's environment to minimize his or her discomfort. For more on strategies for behavioral management, go to pages 103-109.

If anxiety symptoms are severely disruptive, the doctor may prescribe short-term doses of medications that may ease some of these symptoms. These medications include anxiolytics, selective serotonin reuptake inhibitors or antipsychotics (for more information, see pages 109-112). Generally, the main side effect from a course of medication is a feeling of sedation, but other possible side effects may worsen the person's situation. Therefore, medication should be used with caution. In addition, antipsychotics are associated with an increased risk of death when used for behavioral disturbances in older adults with dementia. This is usually as a result of a heart-related event, such as heart failure or sudden death, or as a result of infections, such as pneumonia.

Sleep disorders

Disturbed sleep patterns are common among people with Alzheimer's, particularly in the later stages of the disease. These disturbances take many forms. Some people may sleep more than they ever did before — up to 16 hours a day. Others may sleep less, perhaps only two to four hours at night. Furthermore, the cycle of sleep and wakefulness may be reversed between night and day. Restlessness and nighttime wandering are common symptoms.

Factors that may contribute to excessive sleeping include medication side effects, metabolic problems and boredom. On the other hand, anxiety and depression can contribute to insomnia, as can lack of daytime physical activity, too much napping, certain medications and excessive intake of stimulants such as caffeine. Keeping a person with Alzheimer's occupied and engaged during the day, monitoring napping and caffeine intake, increasing physical activity and maintaining a reasonable bedtime (not too early) may help improve sleep patterns.

Other sleep disorders that commonly affect people with Alzheimer's include sleep apnea, restless leg syndrome and periodic limb movements during sleep. Some people may seem to "act out" their dreams. People with Alzheimer's may snore loudly and experience episodes of snorting or gasping, a creepy-crawly sensation in their legs (especially at night) or nightmares. These signs and symptoms should be discussed with a doctor. Most of these sleep disorders are treatable, and successful treatment can improve cognition, mood and quality of life.

These disturbances often affect the caregiver's sleep patterns as well. If this happens, it's important that the caregiver find alternate ways to obtain necessary rest, so he or she doesn't become sleep deprived. Sleep disturbances often become a decisive factor for placing a person in a nursing home.

Alzheimer's and other forms of dementia

As described previously, Alzheimer's disease sometimes occurs in conjunction with other dementia-causing disorders. This presents a challenge to the doctor attempting a diagnosis. Because treatment options may vary, your doctor will carefully study all of the signs and symptoms and perform various tests in hopes of distinguishing between Alzheimer's and another dementia These include vascular cognitive impairment and dementia with Lewy bodies.

Vascular cognitive impairment

About a quarter of all people with Alzheimer's disease in fact have Alzheimer's combined with another disorder called vascular cognitive impairment, also known as vascular dementia. Vascular cognitive impairment can result from an interruption of blood flow to the brain, either from a blockage of arteries or from a series of strokes. A person's mental capabilities deteriorate step by step with each additional stroke.

Not surprisingly, a major risk factor is a history of strokes. Other risk factors include high blood pressure and high cholesterol levels. Paralysis, vision loss and difficulty with speaking and using language are commonly found in people who have vascular cognitive impairment. Often, the onset of this disorder is sudden and abrupt, but occasionally the disease progresses more slowly, making it difficult to distinguish from Alzheimer's. For more information on vascular cognitive impairment, see Chapter 9.

Dementia with Lewy body and Parkinson's disease

Lewy bodies are abnormal protein deposits in the brain that progressively destroy neurons. When Lewy bodies are widespread throughout the brain, a person may have symptoms similar to those of both Alzheimer's disease and Parkinson's disease. Concentration problems and other cognitive symptoms often appear first. Later, the stiffness and slowness of movement associated with Parkinson's occurs. The person also may experience visual hallucinations. The cause of dementia with Lewy bodies is unknown, but recent studies indicate that it's a common cause of dementia. For more information on DLB, see Chapter 8.

About 20 percent of people with Alzheimer's also have Parkinson's disease. Parkinson's is a crippling illness affecting nerve cells in the parts of the brain that control muscle movements. It's characterized by stiffness of the limbs, tremors, difficulty with walking and speech impairment. Lewy bodies often appear in damaged regions of the brains of people with Parkinson's disease and some people with Alzheimer's also have these particular protein deposits. This suggests a close but still undetermined relationship among all three disorders.

Advancing our understanding

Scientists describe the disease process in stages according to signs and symptoms as Alzheimer's advances through various parts of the brain. The scientists have also identified conditions, including other forms of dementia, which may exist concurrently with Alzheimer's. This knowledge helps determine the treatment for various cognitive and behavioral symptoms of Alzheimer's disease, greatly improving the quality of life for the person with dementia and reducing the workload stress for the caregiver. The subject of the next chapter is the biological basis of this insidious disease, a vital and still unanswered question.

Chapter 5

Biological basis of Alzheimer's

E ver since Alois Alzheimer identified the characteristic plaques and tangles of Alzheimer's disease in the early 20th century, scientists have ardently pursued hundreds of different leads in a quest to understand the destructive nature of the disease. The pace of this research has accelerated in recent years, with scientists gaining valuable insight into the physiological and chemical complexities of the brain.

Investigating the causes of Alzheimer's is like piecing together a jigsaw puzzle. The problem is, there's no guide to show what the finished product will look like. Furthermore, the jumbled pieces seem to come from different and seemingly unrelated puzzles. And no one knows if all the pieces are present and accounted for or if one or two pieces are still missing.

Scientists do know that the disease is very likely caused by a combination of factors. A substantial number of people with Alzheimer's have a family history of dementia, indicating that genes play a role. And some rare forms of Alzheimer's are clearly inherited. But genetic factors aren't the whole story. Researchers are also investigating environmental or lifestyle factors that may contribute to the development of Alzheimer's. Scientists aren't sure how all these elements are related or what other factors are yet to be identified, but a broader perspective is emerging.

Plaques and tangles

A characteristic feature of Alzheimer's disease is the abundance of two kinds of abnormal structures in the brain — amyloid plaques and neurofibrillary tangles. In 1907, Dr. Alois Alzheimer published an account of a woman showing symptoms of severe memory loss and paranoia. An examination of brain tissue following her death revealed large accumulations of these structures.

Plaques and tangles aren't unique to Alzheimer's. They've been observed in other types of dementia. In fact, they can develop in the brain tissue of people who show no symptoms of dementia at all. But in people with Alzheimer's, plaques and tangles occur in far greater number. The focus of much research today is determining how the two are connected to the disease process.

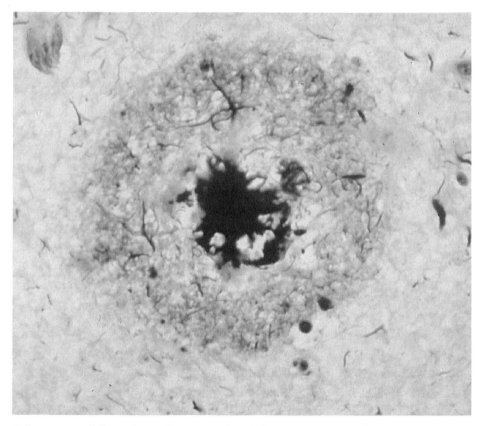

A dense core of tissue lies at the center of amyloid plaques. Surrounding the core is an area of inflammation.

Amyloid plaques

Amyloid plaques are large, undissolvable (insoluble) clumps of tissue found between and around living nerve cells. These plaques consist mainly of a protein called beta-amyloid, mixed with bits of degenerating cellular material and other protein fragments.

Beta-amyloid is, in fact, a protein fragment clipped by enzymes from what's known as the amyloid precursor protein (APP). (See page 83 and page 58 of the Visual Guide for more information on how beta-amyloid fragments are formed.) The normal function of the protein is still uncertain, but studies indicate that APP plays an important role in the growth and maintenance of neurons.

Other types of protein fragments are clipped off of APP, but beta-amyloid appears to be longer and stickier. "Stickier" in this instance refers to the tendency of certain beta-amyloid fragments to agglomerate into a mass and not dissolve, unlike the other kinds of protein fragments.

Based on current research, it appears that the beta-amyloid fragments pass through several stages before forming a plaque. At first a few beta-amyloid fragments clump together and yet are still fairly easy to dissolve. At this stage they're called oligomers (OL-ih-go-murz). But when several oligomers join together, the clumps become ever larger and stickier, forming long fibrillar chains of amyloid fragments. Eventually, accumulations of these chains harden into the insoluble plaques that are characteristic of the disease.

The prevailing theory among scientists is that beta-amyloid is somehow responsible for much of the damage to neurons caused by Alzheimer's. Studies suggest that the processing of beta-amyloid plays a role in various genetic mutations associated with the disease. For example, a mutation of the APP gene — on chromosome 21 — is known to cause Alzheimer's. All known examples of the inherited forms of Alzheimer's disease are accompanied by a large increase in the level of beta-amyloid protein in the brain. In addition, people with Down syndrome — who by the nature of their condition carry three APP genes (instead of the normal two) — frequently develop Alzheimer's later in life.

For a long time, scientists believed that the plaques themselves were toxic to neurons, leading to the cell death. But as more evidence is uncovered regarding the way in which plaques are formed, some scientists are beginning to reconsider this position. They argue that the time when beta-amyloid is most toxic to neurons is in the early stages of plaque formation — in the oligomer stage.

These scientists have given oligomers a special name: amyloid-beta-derived diffusible ligands, or ADDLs for short. Based on various studies, they believe that the ADDLs attack and destroy the brain's synapses — the spaces across which neurons must communicate with one another — resulting in the memory loss and other cognitive impairments that develop in Alzheimer's. By the time large plaques form, the beta-amyloid fragments may have already lost their toxicity and the insoluble clumps are merely inert masses. In other words, the plaques are byproducts of the disease rather than actively participating in its development.

Still, the unanswered question is whether beta-amyloid is a direct cause of cognitive decline. Would removing excess beta-

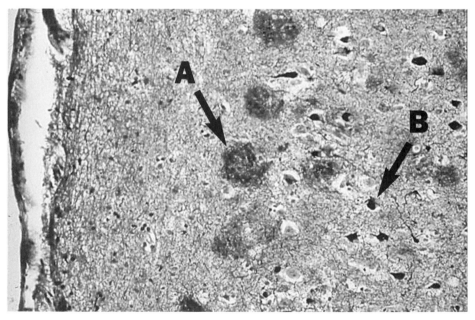

Characteristic features of Alzheimer's

This microphotograph of brain tissue shows the accumulation of beta-amyloid plaques (arrow A) and neurofibrillary tangles (arrow B) in a person with Alzheimer's disease.

amyloid from the brain or halting overproduction of beta-amyloid eliminate the cognitive and behavioral symptoms of AD? Increasingly, researchers are leaning towards the belief that the best opportunity for reversing the disease may be at the oligomer stage, while the agglomerations are small and beta-amyloid fragments still soluble, preventing them from doing irreversible damage.

Neurofibrillary tangles

The other abnormal structures that are so characteristic of Alzheimer's disease are neurofibrillary tangles. The tangles are caused by abnormal processing of a protein called tau (tou) within the cell body. Tau normally helps uphold the structure of a neuron, but as Alzheimer's develops, the protein undergoes chemical changes that cause it to malfunction. Instead of stabilizing the cell's internal structure, tau proteins begin to unravel and clump together, forming tangled masses inside the cell. For more information on this breakdown, see page 59 in the Visual Guide.

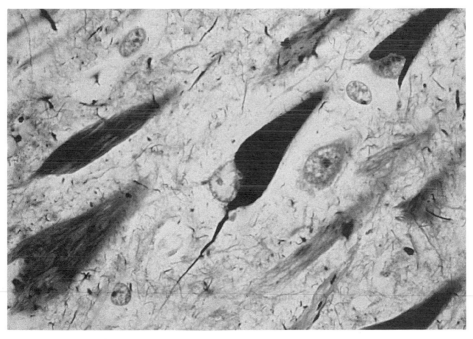

The dark mass on this microphotograph is the collapsed structure of a neuron. Tau protein within the cell has twisted and loosened, undoing the cell structure.

The neurofibrillary tangles have a devastating effect on the structure and function of neurons. They interfere with the transportation of nutrients within the cells and with the transmission of electric impulses to adjoining cells, leading to the collapse of vital cell functions, including intercellular communication.

Some evidence suggests that the production of beta-amyloid protein may stimulate the formation of tangles, perhaps by upsetting calcium levels within the cells. At this point, however, the relationship between beta-amyloid and tau tangles remains unclear.

As with beta-amyloid plaques, scientists continue to debate whether neurofibrillary tangles are a cause of Alzheimer's disease or a result of it. Accumulation of the tangles appears to be closely related to the severity of the dementia symptoms. However, tangles don't appear to necessarily cause neuron death. Some researchers suggest that tangles may be a response to oxidative stress in the brain (see page 87 for more on oxidative stress).

Neurofibrillary tangles can be found in the brain tissue of people with other forms of dementia, including FTDP-17, an inherited form of frontotemporal dementia caused by a mutation of the tau gene on chromosome 17. The effect of this mutation in FTDP-17 is similar to what happens in Alzheimer's — the twisting of tau protein threads and the accumulation of tangles in the cell. Research into other dementias such as these may eventually offer clues to the role tangles play in Alzheimer's disease.

Contributing factors

Researchers are studying alternative explanations for the disease process. Although beta-amyloid aggregation and the formation of tangles may be prominent steps, other changes may occur early in the process that contribute to disease development. These mechanisms include inflammatory response, oxidative stress and cardiovascular events. In fact, some scientists contest that one or more of these factors are a main cause of Alzheimer's and that the plaques and tangles may have formed as an attempt to protect the brain from damage.

Inflammatory response

Inflammation is your body's protective response to injury or infection and a natural part of the healing process. It may involve pain, swelling, heat and redness of the inflamed region. Various studies have observed a certain amount of inflammation in the brain tissue of people with Alzheimer's disease.

What could be causing this phenomenon? Even as beta-amyloid plaques develop in the space between neurons, immune cells (microglia) are going about their normal work of clearing dead cells and other waste products from the brain. Scientists speculate that the microglia identify plaques as foreign substances in the body and are trying to destroy them, triggering the inflammatory response. Or the microglia may be trying to remove damaged neurons. Or the microglia may be activating compounds that cause inflammation — these include the protein interleukin-1, the enzyme COX-2 and a group of proteins, known as complement, which take action against cells marked by microglia for removal.

Although researchers believe inflammation develops before the plaques have fully formed, they aren't sure how this occurrence relates to the disease process. There's also debate about whether inflammation has a damaging effect on neurons or whether it's in any way beneficial for clearing away the plaques.

Oxidative stress

Oxidative stress occurs when there's damage to the mitochondria, structures that are the energy factories of a cell. Damaged mitochondria tend to overproduce highly reactive molecules called free radicals. Normally, free radicals perform a number of useful tasks, but too many free radicals become a problem. They overwhelm and damage the cell, resulting in tissue breakdown and damage to DNA. Normal aging can lead to a buildup of free radicals and to oxidative stress, as can various disease-related factors.

What causes the oxidative stress? Evidence suggests that beta-amyloid aggregation and possibly the inflammatory response may play roles. Signs of oxidative stress have been observed in the brains of people with Alzheimer's, particularly in the late stages when plaques and tangles are plentiful.

On the other hand, oxidative stress may occur before the formation of plaques and tangles. There are indications of oxidative stress in the earliest stages of the disease, which may even lead to the formation of beta-amyloid fragments and neurofibrillary tangles. Some researchers argue that plaques and tangles are formed as protective measure against oxidative stress.

Still other researchers contend that a chronic state of low-level oxidative stress, when combined with certain abnormalities in the regulation of cell growth, may be sufficient to trigger the beginnings of damaging changes to the brain's neurons.

Regardless of whether oxidative stress is an initiator or a result of neuron damage, most researchers agree that it likely plays a vital role in the disease process.

Cardiovascular risk factors

Scientists have long known that factors such as high blood pressure and high cholesterol can severely damage blood vessels, leading to increased risk of heart disease and stroke.

But factors such as high blood pressure and high cholesterol can also affect blood vessels in the brain (cerebrovascular disease), sometimes generating sufficient damage — through strokes or an insufficient supply of nutrients — to cause dementia. Dementia caused by cerebrovascular disease is generally referred to as vascular cognitive impairment.

Recent studies suggest that these same factors may also increase the likelihood that you'll develop Alzheimer's disease. For example, increased concentrations of cholesterol in the brain appear to increase the production of beta-amyloid. Scientists continue to actively pursue clues to the exact relationship between cardiovascular risk factors and Alzheimer's (See Chapter 13).

What's becoming apparent is that Alzheimer's disease and vascular cognitive impairment frequently occur at the same time in the same person and that when they do the symptoms of dementia appear to be compounded — being more severe than when either condition occurs alone. This suggests that Alzheimer's symptoms are more likely to develop if strokes or damage to blood vessels in the brain has taken place.

Other risk factors

Research suggests that a number of other factors are connected to the Alzheimer's disease process in some way. Factors such as age are definitely established, and others are still under investigation.

Age. The total number of Alzheimer's cases (prevalence) rises dramatically with age, doubling every five years after the age of 65. The number of new AD cases reported (incidence) rises in similar fashion with age. Some researchers speculate that Alzheimer's is an inevitable consequence of aging. In other words, if you live long enough you will eventually develop the disease. However, the fact that many older adults, including people in their 90s or 100s, still display sharp memories and cognitive skills contradicts this theory.

Other scientists postulate that Alzheimer's develops within a specific age range and that an increase in the prevalence of AD levels off around the age of 95. A growing consensus is that although Alzheimer's is not a normal part of aging, the effects of aging may strengthen its development.

Sex. Studies based on the prevalence of Alzheimer's show that more women have dementia than men. This can be explained, at least in part, by women generally living longer than men and perhaps even surviving longer with dementia. Combined data from a number of European studies spanning the years 1988 to 1996 suggests that women also may have a slightly higher risk of developing dementia, particularly Alzheimer's. Scientists don't understand the reason for this finding, but possibilities may include biological differences. The studies have also been questioned for bias in diagnostic testing or for an unequal distribution of risk factors among males and females.

Education. Several studies have detected a correlation between a low level of education and higher risk of dementia and, conversely, a high level of education and lower dementia risk.

The findings from a project known as the Nun Study support the idea that education may protect individuals from developing Alzheimer's disease. The researchers examined autobiographies written by a group of nuns at the time of their entrance into a Milwaukee convent. The average age of these new entrants was 22. The essays were measured for their density of ideas — the average number of ideas per 10 words — and their grammatical complexity. The nuns had also willed their brains to research with the intention of an autopsy being performed after they died. Surprisingly, the researchers found that 90 percent of the nuns who had a low density of ideas in their autobiographies also showed evidence of accumulated neurofibrillary tangles in their brains. Those nuns who had had a high density of ideas in their autobiographies had very few tangles at the time of autopsy.

Subsequent studies mostly confirm the notion that low levels of education might be a risk factor for the later development of Alzheimer's. Some researchers theorize that the more you use your brain, the more synapses you create between neurons. Theoretically, this provides a greater reserve of brainpower from which you may draw on to compensate for later neuron loss. It remains unclear, however, whether lower education and less mental activity create a risk of Alzheimer's or if it's simply harder to detect Alzheimer's in people who exercise their minds frequently or who have a higher education level.

Head injury. The observation that some ex-boxers eventually develop dementia raises the question of whether serious traumatic injury to the head (for example, a prolonged loss of consciousness) may be a risk factor of Alzheimer's. Several studies indicate a significant link between the two, especially among men. Other studies find only a slight, nonsignificant correlation between head trauma and Alzheimer's. The debate is still ongoing, but one of the theories is that head injury may interact with a gene linked to Alzheimer's disease.

Genetic factors affecting Alzheimer's disease

Certain genetic mutations — defects in single genes or in sections of chromosomes — are known to cause a small number of inherited forms of Alzheimer's disease. These genes include the APP gene and the presenilin genes, presenilin 1 (PS1) and presenilin 2 (PS2). The locations of these genes in human DNA are indicated in the chart on page 92.

> **Amyloid precursor protein**
>
> Amyloid precursor protein (APP) is sometimes called a membrane protein because it becomes lodged like a pin stuck in a cushion — partly inside and partly outside the cell membrane, the thin outer covering of a cell. In this position, APP is clipped off outside the membrane by an enzyme, another type of protein that speeds up reactions.
>
> Many of the APP clippings dissolve fairly easily and are removed from the brain eventually as waste. Certain other clippings are longer, "stickier" fragments that don't dissolve so easily. These longer beta-amyloid fragments agglomerate with other waste products into dense masses that harden to form the Alzheimer's plaques. For a visual image of this process, see page 58 in the Visual Guide.
>
> Scientists have identified mutations of the APP gene on chromosome 21 that cause a rare form of Alzheimer's disease. These mutations are located on part of the APP that's sticking outside the cell membrane and close to the clipping sites. This may mean the mutations play a role in the formation of more beta-amyloid or more of the "stickier" beta-amyloid fragments. Either case would lead to the creation of more plaques.

People who inherit one of these rare mutations usually begin to experience symptoms before the age of 65 (a condition known as early-onset Alzheimer's). Symptoms of and treatment for this form of Alzheimer's are generally no different from the noninherited forms of Alzheimer's. A parent who has any one of these known mutations has a high chance of passing it on to his or her child — each child has a 50 percent chance of inheriting the abnormal gene and developing the disease.

Something all genetic mutations known to cause Alzheimer's have in common is the abnormal processing of the amyloid precursor protein and excessive production of beta-amyloid fragments. In fact, scientists think that the presenilin genes PS1 and PS2 are most likely forms of one of the enzymes that helps create the stickier and more toxic version of beta-amyloid.

Genes associated with Alzheimer's

Gene	Chromosome
Amyloid precursor protein (APP)	21
Presenilin 1 (PS1)	14
Presenilin 2 (PS2)	1
Apolipoprotein E (APOE ε4)	19

Apolipoprotein E

In addition to finding genetic mutations that cause Alzheimer's, scientists have identified a normal gene — the apolipoprotein E (APOE) gene — that may increase a person's risk of the more common form of Alzheimer's that develops after age 65 (a condition known as late-onset Alzheimer's).

Before being linked to Alzheimer's disease, the APOE gene was already known in the medical community for its role in carrying blood cholesterol through the body. There are three alleles, or variants, of APOE — named ε2, ε3 and ε4.

Unlike the APP, PS1 and PS2 genes, it's not a mutation of APOE that plays a role in Alzheimer's but one of these naturally occurring variants of the gene — the ε4 allele. And while inheriting one of the APP, PS1 and PS2 mutations is certain to lead to early-onset Alzheimer's, inheriting one or two of the APOE ε4 alleles doesn't guarantee a person will develop Alzheimer's. But having the APOE ε4 allele does greatly increase your chance of getting the disease. For example, a person with two ε4 alleles has a 9- to 10-fold increased risk. This risk appears to peak around 70 years of age and in later years levels off. Having the ε4 allele may also lower the age of disease onset — usually several years earlier than non-APOE ε4-related forms of Alzheimer's.

Surprisingly, the APOE ε2 variant may have a protective effect against Alzheimer's disease. This is suggested by the fact that people who carry a mutated APP gene — a known cause of early-onset Alzheimer's — and the APOE ε2 allele have failed to develop dementia as expected.

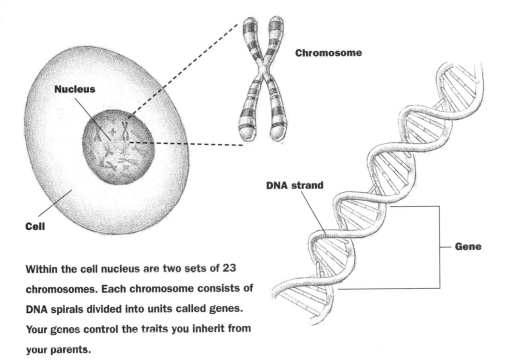

Within the cell nucleus are two sets of 23 chromosomes. Each chromosome consists of DNA spirals divided into units called genes. Your genes control the traits you inherit from your parents.

Research indicates that the APOE ε4 allele is associated with an increase in the amount of beta-amyloid in the brain, but exactly how this happens is under debate. Some researchers suspect that unlike the ε3 and ε2 alleles, the ε4 allele simply is ineffective at dissolving beta-amyloid from the brain.

A complicated process

The emerging picture of Alzheimer's disease involves an intricate process that may include beta-amyloid aggregation into plaques, neurofibrillary tangles, inflammation, oxidative stress, cellular imbalance, genetic susceptibility and other as yet unknown risk factors. The difficulty of predicting who will or will not develop Alzheimer's may remain a characteristic of the disease in itself. This means that although researchers may identify common physiological pathways for Alzheimer's to develop in most people, its occurrence in specific individuals may be precipitated by different combinations of genetic and environmental triggers.

What about genetic screening?

Although genetic screening kits are available for presenilin 1 (PS1) mutations and for the apolipoprotein E (APOE) allele e4, most Alzheimer's specialists don't routinely recommend these tests. However, if a person is exhibiting early symptoms of dementia and another close family member has already been diagnosed with early-onset Alzheimer's, screening tests for a PS1 mutation may be useful for the diagnosis.

Most researchers agree that screening for the APOE e4 gene has little predictive value. That's because having this gene doesn't mean a person will get Alzheimer's, and not having the gene doesn't mean you won't get the disease. If preventive treatment ever becomes available, this test will be more useful to a wider number of people.

Although key factors in the disease process are being revealed, many important questions about these factors remain unanswered. What roles do plaques and tangles play in the damage to and eventual death of neurons? How are inflammation, oxidative stress and cardiovascular risk factors involved in the process? What environmental factors, if any, affect the onset and progression of the disease? Will new treatments targeted at eliminating plaques and tangles also address the cognitive and physical symptoms of AD? What is it that allows some people in their 90s or 100s to retain their memory and intellectual skills? These are the issues that scientists continue to pursue in the quest to understand Alzheimer's.

Chapter 6

Treatment of Alzheimer's

lthough scientists around the world are working intently to develop therapies that can halt or delay Alzheimer's disease, and possibly even prevent it, no such therapy is currently available. The treatment strategies in practice today are focused on managing symptoms of the disease. For example, treatment aims to help maintain memory, reduce anxieties, raise spirits, relieve health concerns and encourage alertness during waking hours or sleep during the night. But it will not stop the disease.

Treatment is most often a combination of drug therapies and personal care. Drug therapies range from medications developed specifically for treating the cognitive symptoms of Alzheimer's to drugs in general use in the mental health field, such as antidepressants and antipsychotics. Personal care is administered by caregivers and specialists in a variety of settings.

Working toward treatment goals

Living with a disease such as Alzheimer's can be a challenge that stretches the courage, fortitude, patience, creativity and adaptive skills of everyone involved. Whether it's the person with the disease or other family members or the primary caregiver, the stress placed on individuals is intense and the demands vary widely. Coping requires trust and honesty among individuals dealing with a host of complex personal issues.

The one constant you must depend on is preparedness for change. Symptoms change or intensify as the disease progresses. In response, the types and combinations of treatment and care will need to be adapted, strengthened or remade to meet different goals. What worked in the mild stage of Alzheimer's may no longer be effective for the moderate and severe stages.

In recognizing the difficult challenge that Alzheimer's disease presents, you also must recognize that you don't have to face this challenge alone. More and more, experts and health care professionals understand and emphasize the need for team effort — a team that includes the caregiver, doctors, nurses, social workers, clinicians, friends, family and, most importantly, the person with Alzheimer's. One of the benefits of the increasing national focus on Alzheimer's disease is the growing number of resources available to people with the condition and to their caregivers.

If you or someone you know has received a diagnosis of Alzheimer's, here are three key guidelines to remember:

Know your resources

To make use of the resources available, you need to know where to find them. The Alzheimer's Association is a key source of information and may be able to refer you to additional local resources. With chapters throughout the United States, the Alzheimer's Association can help you find specialists, support groups, in-home services, respite care, financial planners and assisted-living facilities. At the back of this book, you'll find a list of organizations, including the Alzheimer's Association, that may be helpful to contact.

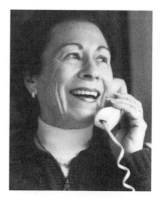

Ask for help

Many people dealing with a dementing disorder, whether it's the person with the disease or the caregiver, find it difficult to ask for help. They often feel that because they're independent-minded adults, they should be able to handle the pressures on their own. This mind-set all too frequently makes the problems worse.

For a person with early-stage Alzheimer's, it can be frightening to admit that you have the disease — which may certainly make you more reluctant to seek help. But at this emotionally fragile time when you're coming to terms with the disease, it's important to remain connected to family and friends. If you falter, they can be there to provide support.

If you're the caregiver, wearing yourself out to the point of exhaustion is not beneficial to you or your loved one. To be able to provide care for others, you must first care for yourself physically and emotionally. This happens by enlisting the help of family members and friends, obtaining advice from experts and thoughtfully addressing problems with the resources at hand.

Don't give up

Just because there's no cure for Alzheimer's right now doesn't mean that you shouldn't seek treatment for the disease. There's a lot you can do to ease symptoms, strengthen emotions, raise spirits and improve the quality of life for everyone involved. But it takes commitment and persistence.

Although Alzheimer's disease will bring dramatic changes to your life and that of your family, remember that there will continue to be good moments and bad moments and even, very likely, humorous moments. So, when possible, step back from the immediate demands of living and coping. Focus your mind on something else — enjoy a morning cup of coffee or watch a favorite movie. Give yourself a moment to breathe. Short respites like these will help keep you going.

The three guidelines described above can help you actively participate with your doctor and a health care team to achieve the treatment goals. Access to a full arsenal of therapies may put the manageable aspects of the disease, for a time at least, under your control. And applying all you've learned about Alzheimer's will assist you or a loved one in facing the challenges of the disease with dignity and grace.

Medications for cognitive symptoms

As discussed in Chapter 4, one of the main neurotransmitters in the brain that's affected by Alzheimer's disease is acetylcholine. Scientists know that levels of acetylcholine drop sharply in people with Alzheimer's — a drop caused at least in part by an enzyme known as acetylcholinesterase (as-uh-tul-ko-li-NES-tuh-ras). Based on this knowledge, scientists have developed drugs to keep, or inhibit, the acetylcholinesterase from acting on acetylcholine. Most of the drugs currently approved by the Food and Drug Administration (FDA) for treating the cognitive symptoms of Alzheimer's work in this manner. Thus, the drugs as a group are called cholinesterase (ko-lin-ES-tur-ays) inhibitors.

Acetylcholine: The thoughtful messenger

Acetylcholine is one of the principal chemical messengers within your body, occurring in both your central and peripheral nervous systems. It controls muscle contractions and hormone secretion and also plays a key role — if still not completely understood — in thinking and memory skills.

In the 1970s, neuroscientists became aware of a dramatic drop in the level of acetylcholine in the brains of people with Alzheimer's disease. Since then, much research has been focused on this neurotransmitter. Scientists have learned that the acetylcholine deficit is related directly to the severity of dementia. This evidence has inspired therapies designed to alter the levels of acetylcholine in the brain in hopes that this action would improve the symptoms of Alzheimer's.

Although scientists are still not sure of the exact role acetylcholine plays in thinking and memory, most agree that it's involved in what's called selective attention. This term refers to the way your brain filters incoming information and processes some messages while ignoring others — essential in starting the memory process. Some researchers speculate that a shortage of acetylcholine also may have a tremendous impact on conscious awareness as well as on memory retrieval.

Until recently, three cholinesterase inhibitors were the only drugs approved for the treatment of Alzheimer's. But in October 2003, the FDA approved the drug memantine (Namenda), a new class of medication specifically intended for use at the moderate and severe stages of Alzheimer's. Memantine seems to slow the loss of many routine skills necessary for daily living, such as dressing, eating and going to the bathroom.

Cholinesterase inhibitors

Currently, cholinesterase inhibitors are used only in the mild to moderate stages of Alzheimer's. During these stages, the inhibitors play a valuable role in managing the disease. They not only stabilize cognitive functions such as memory, judgment and attention, but also seem to have a positive effect on behavior.

After the moderate stage, the drugs appear to lose much of their effectiveness and the cognitive decline resumes, although some evidence suggests that continued use of these drugs may help improve psychiatric and behavioral symptoms even in more advanced stages and may help delay the need for a nursing home. The long-term effects of these medications aren't known, but studies are under way to follow their full course.

Available cholinesterase inhibitors are donepezil, rivastigmine and galantamine. Although these medications are generally well tolerated, gastrointestinal problems are common side effects. These include nausea, diarrhea, stomach pain, loss of appetite and vomiting. The side effects often go away with time. Tacrine (Cognex) is an older cholinesterase inhibitor that's no longer used because of severe side effects.

Donepezil. Approved by the FDA in 1996, donepezil (Aricept) is the most commonly prescribed cholinesterase inhibitor. It comes in tablet form and is taken orally once a day. The doctor may start someone with a dose of 5 milligrams (mg) and then increase the dose to 10 mg if the person tolerates the drug well. In clinical trials people with Alzheimer's who took donepezil did better on memory and reasoning assessments than did those who were given an inactive substance (placebo). One of the benefits of donepezil is that its side effects are generally mild.

Rivastigmine. This drug is similar to donepezil in its action. Rivastigmine (Exelon), however, is taken orally twice a day and comes in capsule or liquid form. Total dosages can range from 6 mg to 12 mg a day. Higher doses of rivastigmine may be more effective than lower doses but also cause more severe side effects. A person will probably start out at a low dose, which may be increased gradually over time. This minimizes discomfort and allows time for the person's body to adjust to the drug. Taking the medication with food may help as well.

Galantamine. Galantamine (Razadyne, formerly Reminyl), the newest cholinesterase inhibitor on the market, improves both cognition and behavior. Long-term effects have not been studied, but it was well tolerated during clinical trials. Galantamine comes in tablet form, and the dosage is increased gradually, to no more than 12 mg twice a day. A new formulation is available for once-a-day dosing. Side effects are usually mild, similar to those of donepezil.

People who are taking a cholinesterase inhibitor often will wonder if the medication is doing any good. They're tempted to stop taking the medication if they don't see immediate benefits. But remember that these drugs are designed to maintain cognitive functions, which are not always easy to check and assess when there's change. Some people who stop taking an inhibitor abruptly experience a dramatic drop in their functional abilities.

How long treatment with cholinesterase inhibitors should continue is uncertain. Most clinical trials of these drugs have lasted only six months but a few trials lasting a year have shown continued benefit in taking an inhibitor. Usually, the period of treatment lasts for about three to five years until symptoms become severe and there's little response if any to the drug.

Currently, there's no evidence to suggest that one cholinesterase inhibitor is better than another. Based on the family's preferences, a doctor might switch prescriptions at some point if a person has an allergic reaction to a drug or cannot tolerate the drug's side effects.

Scientists are testing whether such drugs are helpful for mild cognitive impairment (MCI) — considered an early transition stage between normal cognition and Alzheimer's. A large trial of the cholinesterase inhibitor donepezil among people with MCI found that it did slow the progression to dementia but only temporarily (for more on this trial, see Chapter 11).

Preliminary studies of galantamine in people with MCI showed no real cognitive benefits or any indication of preventing the progression from MCI to Alzheimer's. Unfortunately, the researchers also observed a higher number of deaths among the people receiving galantamine as opposed to participants receiving a placebo. Further research is ongoing on the effectiveness of cholinesterase inhibitors as a treatment for MCI.

Memantine

Memantine (Namenda) is the first drug of its type to be approved for Alzheimer's in the United States. It's officially classified as an N-methyl-D-aspartate (NMDA) receptor antagonist. What this means is that it works by regulating the interactions of glutamate — a neurotransmitter involved in memory and learning — and NMDA neuron receptors — a receptor being the part of the neuron that receives an impulse.

If you'll recall, neurons communicate with one another when an impulse triggers the release of neurotransmitters into the synapse — the space between two adjoining nerve cells. The neurotransmitters released from one cell bind to specific receptors on the next cell, allowing the impulse to be passed on.

Normally, the neurotransmitter glutamate binds to NMDA receptors in a cell for the purposes of memory storage. But too much glutamate can overstimulate the receptors. This excessive activity is thought to be one of the mechanisms causing nerve cell degeneration in dementia.

Memantine works by blocking the NMDA receptors so that glutamate can't bind to them. This reduces the excess amount of glutamate-induced activity amongst neurons and protects them from damaging side effects.

Originally approved for use in Europe, the drug was also approved in the United States after clinical trials showed it to be safe and modestly effective for Alzheimer's disease. In general, memantine appears to improve or at least temporarily stabilize a person's behavior and ability to function in daily life.

Memantine is taken orally. Like other Alzheimer's drugs, it's usually started at a low dose and then increased to a recommended dose of 20 mg a day (10 mg twice a day). Side effects may include headache, constipation, confusion, dizziness and seizures.

Because cholinesterase inhibitors and memantine differ markedly in their actions, a doctor may prescribe a cholinesterase inhibitor with memantine in order for the person to get the benefits of both.

Vitamin E

Although the jury is still out on whether vitamin E improves cognition in people with Alzheimer's disease — vitamin E is thought to reduce the amount of oxidative stress that may contribute to the disease process — many doctors prescribe high-dose supplements of the vitamin along with cholinesterase inhibitors or memantine. A study conducted in 1997 reported that vitamin E produced a significant time delay in the development of severe dementia, placement in a nursing home, impairment of daily living skills, and death.

Nonmedication therapy for cognitive symptoms

Aside from medications, memory aids can help a person with Alzheimer's supplement cognitive losses and maintain a degree of independence. You can do this by writing down information and keeping it in visible places, along with well-placed clocks and calendars. Create a list of the day's activities, including specific instructions for tasks such as getting dressed and preparing food. Make a list of important phone numbers. Label drawers with their respective contents and label entrances to different rooms with their functions, for example, "bathroom" and "bedroom." For more memory tips, see Chapter 12.

For a caregiver, as the disease progresses, it may be more important to provide reassurance rather than trying to reorient the person to the current time or place or the real version of events. If your loved one becomes worried about a family member or friend who is no longer living, for example, it's often more comforting to reassure him or her that everything is OK than to insist upon a recognition of reality.

Recently, however, an analysis of several vitamin E studies revealed that high doses of vitamin E may slightly increase a person's risk of death, mostly in people with heart disease. This finding was not reported in the initial 1997 trial that gave such positive indications. At this time, if a person with Alzheimer's also has heart disease, the doctor may refrain from prescribing vitamin supplements to limit risk. Additional studies are needed to determine whether lower doses of vitamin E are beneficial to people with Alzheimer's who don't have heart disease.

Strategies for behavioral symptoms

As Alzheimer's disease progresses, extreme changes in mood and behavior become common. This may result from the damage to neurons and cell communication in the brain. It may also be a result of damage to the limbic system — the part of the brain associated with feelings and emotions. Many abnormal behaviors are an unfortunate outgrowth of the individual's progressively worsening impairments to cognition — inability to remember things, to reason with others and to resolve problems. Challenging behaviors often associated with Alzheimer's include:

- Aggression
- Agitation
- Delusions
- Hallucinations
- Resisting help
- Suspiciousness or paranoia
- Sleep disturbances
- Wandering

It's important to remember that someone with Alzheimer's is gradually losing his or her language skills and ability to communicate. These behaviors may be the only way that person can express discomfort, stress and frustration. Even if speech remains intact, there may be difficulties in forming and expressing thoughts correctly. The behaviors listed above may be the only means to communicate urgent feelings and needs.

Without much thought, it would be easy to label a challenging behavior, or even the person with Alzheimer's who displays that behavior, as "bad" or a "problem." It's important to resist labeling for two major reasons. For one thing, troublesome behaviors are rarely acted out on purpose or manipulatively — they arise from the disease process. For another thing, these labels create the expectation that there is "good" behavior — an expectation that the person may not be able to meet. Unfulfilled expectations may foster a sense of futility, resignation or anger.

Following are strategies that may prove helpful in dealing with challenging behaviors.

Identify secondary causes

Many times behavioral problems occur not because of cognitive impairment caused by the disease but because of secondary issues. Health, psychological, environmental and social factors all can have a profound effect on a person with dementia. Problems stemming from these factors are termed excess disability — which means the problems occur in addition to the signs and symptoms caused directly by Alzheimer's. If these problems can be identified, a caregiver may focus on eliminating, modifying or preventing the aggravating factors. Therefore, when addressing behavioral issues associated with dementia, it's helpful to consider a wide range of factors that could be contributing to the problem.

Distinguishing between the symptoms caused by Alzheimer's and those by a secondary source can be challenging. Possible indications that there's a nondementia-related cause include:

- A behavior that's brand new
- A sudden, noticeable decline in function
- A conspicuous worsening of confusion

If one of these indicators occur, you may need to consult your doctor. Treatment of a secondary problem often results in improved behavior, even though the improvement may be temporary.

Health problems. A physical problem can bring out complaints from just about anyone. Someone with Alzheimer's disease is no exception, but because the person may have difficulty communicating verbally what's wrong, he or she may exhibit behavioral problems. Challenging behavior can arise from pain, hunger, fatigue, medication side effects, dehydration, constipation or an illness such as a respiratory condition or type of infection. Impaired hearing or vision can further isolate the person and become a source of hallucinations and delusions. If you suspect an underlying health problem in your loved one, talk to your doctor about ways to treat or manage the problem.

Psychological issues. Anxiety and depression are common among people with Alzheimer's disease. Anxiety is often expressed by excessive concern over upcoming events or by wandering, screaming or acting aggressively. Feelings of anxiety can be caused by a number of factors, including illness, abuse, loss of a loved one or frustration over cognitive decline. Feelings of depression may translate into periods of tearfulness, thoughts of worthlessness and concerns about being a burden on the family. Depression may also come across as a worsening of thinking and reasoning skills, and result in social withdrawal, weight loss, disruptive behavior and decreased functional abilities.

Fortunately, both anxiety and depression are treatable (see Chapter 4). Obtaining a diagnosis from the doctor can lead to more realistic expectations and better knowledge of how to communicate with and care for the person with Alzheimer's.

Support groups and professional counseling may help people in the early stages of Alzheimer's who are depressed but still communicating well. Physical exercise and planned activities also may alleviate symptoms of anxiety or depression by providing a sense of purpose, self-worth and accomplishment.

It's important for a person with Alzheimer's to avoid caffeine and alcohol, as these substances act as stimulants. If symptoms of anxiety and depression are severe, treatment may include anti-anxiety (anxiolytic) or antidepressant medications.

Environmental factors. Understimulation or overstimulation within a person's surroundings can have a significant impact on his or her behavior. With nothing to do, a person with Alzheimer's may become bored or restless and resort to wandering or yelling to release frustration. On the other hand, multiple or unnecessary stimuli may confuse and overwhelm the person.

Television shows may be misunderstood or mistaken for reality by the person with AD, resulting in frightened or angry reactions. The disembodied voices coming from radios, paging systems or people conversing out of sight also may contribute to confusion, paranoia, agitation, hallucinations and delusions. Creating a safe, serene and predictable environment can provide a sense of familiarity and comfort for the person with Alzheimer's and reduce the risk of disruptive behavior.

Social isolation. Although a person with Alzheimer's experiences a progressive loss of his or her ability to communicate with others, the person will still retain basic human needs to belong, to be loved and to feel useful. Social isolation can lead to depression and anxiety as well as to any number of unwanted behaviors, including agitation, delusions, aggression and wandering. Providing the person with a variety of simple, routine social opportunities can help prevent the feeling of isolation.

Stay engaged

One way to improve quality of life and prevent challenging behaviors from developing is to make sure the person with Alzheimer's is involved in daily activities and routine tasks. Staying occupied can make the person feel that he or she is needed and participating in the normal rhythms of life.

At the same time, it's important to involve the person at a level in which he or she can feel comfortable of achieving success. What a person with dementia is able to accomplish may vary from day to day. Sometimes, tasks such as getting dressed may present little problem and at other times they will seem overwhelming.

Try to break each task into simple steps, limit choices and allow extra time for the person to accomplish the chore. Rushing the process or pressuring the person to remember may only cause frustration and panic. Argument and accusation are usually counterproductive. More details on assisting a loved one in everyday tasks can be found in the Action Guide for Caregivers.

A 1999 study funded by the National Institute of Nursing Research revealed that allowing people with Alzheimer's to accomplish as much on their own as possible reinforced their existing skills and helped maintain their independence. For example, even though the time needed for participants to finish dressing on their own nearly doubled, disruptive behaviors decreased. At the same time, requests for assistance increased.

Involvement in recreational activities also can help relieve behavioral symptoms. Enjoyable pastimes may include singing or listening to music, painting, playing board games, walking or reading. The type of activity and the way it's performed is less important than the level of fulfillment and social interaction that the activity provides. For example, the delight your loved one may derive from being able to read a few sentences from the newspaper is far greater than whether he or she is holding the paper properly and able to read the entire article.

Join, validate, distract

As the disease progresses, people with Alzheimer's tend to forget or lose their comprehension of the present reality and revert to a reality they've retained in their remote memory, such as when they were a child or a young adult. In their minds, their parents may still be alive, their children may be toddlers or they may wish to see or talk with a long deceased spouse. If they're confronted with present reality, they may respond by becoming upset, aggressive, withdrawn or even more determined to pursue an intended, albeit irrational, course of action.

In such circumstances, it may be more constructive to join the person's reality, validate how the person is feeling and eventually find a way to distract the person with another thought or activity. Generally, it's best to respond as though you believe what the person has said is true. Then give an explanation that makes sense in that context.

For example, you might tell your mother that her parents aren't home because they've gone to visit relatives, or that there's no need to go to school today because it's Saturday. This may make you feel like you're manipulating and lying. But with the changes to reality in your mother's mind, your goal is not to make sure she's factually correct. It's more important to comfort her. Frame your response in a way that she can understand and feel reassured by.

Keep in mind that the emotions that the person expresses are very real, even if the reasons behind these emotions aren't logical. Some people in the early stages of Alzheimer's disease report that they feel people no longer take them seriously. Show your loved one that you're listening by making eye contact and giving feedback. Validate his or her feelings by acknowledging you recognize the emotions and concerns.

Find activities that distract your loved one's attention elsewhere and focuses it on something positive. If your mother is upset because she thinks she needs to go home and care for her young children, for example, you can join her reality and acknowledge how upset she is without making light of her distress. Provide an explanation that makes sense — for example, the children are at a birthday party having a great time and won't be home for several hours. Then distract her with an activity such as baking cookies or listening to favorite music.

Anticipate potential problems

Heading off problems before they occur can also be an effective way for a caregiver to manage behavior. This is sometimes called the ABC method, where *A* stands for antecedent, *B* for behavior and *C* for consequence. Most behaviors have an antecedent or cause. And behaviors generally lead to some type of consequence. Negative consequences can be difficult to resolve.

Antecedent
Car parked in driveway

↓

Behavior
Outburst of anger

↓

Consequence
Calming and distracting your loved one

As a caregiver, you may be tempted to concentrate mainly on the consequences of a behavior because these demand your immediate attention. But a little forethought can go a long way. By addressing the antecedent first, you may be able to avert both the behavior and the consequences.

For example, seeing a car parked in the driveway may provoke outbursts of anger in a person with Alzheimer's — the person may be reminded that he or she can no longer drive. And because it's likely that you're still able to drive, the anger is directed at you.

Attempts to soothe and distract the person may seem futile. Using the ABC approach, you might decide to park the car at another location and out of sight. This addresses the cause of the outburst and eliminates needless frustration and wasted energy.

Not all behaviors have antecedents that are so readily apparent. But whether a behavior has a clear antecedent or not, being adaptive is an important part of caregiving. With wandering, for example, you may wish to simply go along with the behavior and not worry about antecedents. If the behavior is relatively benign and can be done in a safe place, such as pacing in an enclosed yard or an open room, it may be an appropriate outlet for feelings that otherwise could be expressed in a threatening manner. Be creative. See what works and what doesn't work. And go easy on yourself. If an approach isn't successful one day, keep in mind that you're doing your best. Simply try something else the next day.

Medication therapies for behavioral symptoms

Sometimes, behavioral therapy and social interaction aren't enough to soothe the challenging behavior or alleviate the symptoms of depression or anxiety. To help, your doctor may prescribe medications that can improve the behavioral symptoms.

Unfortunately, there's no medication that can treat all of the behavioral symptoms associated with Alzheimer's. Although medications such as the ones described on the following pages may be of some benefit, they're often used as a second line of defense. That's because these drugs can intensify the cognitive losses of dementia — such as memory loss — and their side effects are generally more severe in older adults.

As a result, it's important to discuss with your doctor and weigh the risks and benefits of a drug before starting to take it. In general, these drugs are best when used only when necessary and for a short period of time.

Some evidence from research suggests that cholinesterase inhibitors may improve behavioral as well as cognitive symptoms. If a person with Alzheimer's isn't already taking a cholinesterase inhibitor, a doctor may recommend one of these drugs before pre-scribing one of the medications that follow.

Antipsychotics

Antipsychotics, also called neuroleptics, may be used to treat chal-lenging behaviors such as aggression, delusions and hallucinations. Antipsychotics are divided into two major groups: conventional and atypical. Both groups work by blocking certain neurotransmit-ter receptors, particularly dopamine, in the hopes of regulating feel-ings and emotions.

Conventional antipsychotics are limited in use for Alzheimer's because their side effects — muscle spasms, rigidity, tremor, gait disturbance and sedation — tend to be severe and typically out-weigh any benefits they may provide.

Atypical antipsychotics are usually the medication of choice for the treatment of agitation or psychosis. In addition to regulating dopamine, they also act on serotonin, a neurotransmitter that affects mood and anxiety. This may be a reason why these medica-tions generally have fewer of the above-mentioned side effects than conventional antipsychotics.

However, antipsychotics, when used to treat behavioral symp-toms in older adults, have been found to increase a person's risk of premature death, usually as a result of a heart-related event or as a result of infection such as pneumonia. The pros and cons of taking the drug must be carefully considered — behaviors can be danger-ous, too — whenever antipsychotics are being considered.

In addition, atypical antipsychotics can raise a person's blood sugar levels to abnormally high levels (hyperglycemia), which can lead to diabetes. Some experts recommend regular screening for diabetes in people who take atypical antipsychotics.

Antipsychotics also block acetylcholine receptors, which are already in short supply in a person with Alzheimer's. This action tends to accelerate cognitive decline.

Commonly prescribed antipsychotic drugs include:
- Olanzapine (Zyprexa)
- Risperidone (Risperdal)
- Quetiapine (Seroquel)

Mood stabilizers

Although not as commonly prescribed as atypical antipsychotics, mood stabilizers (or anticonvulsants) may also be used to treat hostility or aggression. They're not always recommended, however, as there's not much evidence to support their effectiveness, and side effects such as sedation can be severe. These drugs include:

- Divalproex (Depakote)
- Carbamazepine (Tegretol)

Anxiolytics

Symptoms of anxiety may be relieved with anxiolytic (ang-zee-oe-LIT-ik) agents. These medications generally are recommended only for occasional or short-term use. Side effects include sleepiness, decreased learning and memory, dizziness and loss of coordination (which may increase the risk of falls), and possibly even more agitation. Anxiolytics include:

- Lorazepam (Ativan)
- Oxazepam (Serax)
- Buspirone (Buspar)

Antidepressants

If a person with Alzheimer's also receives a diagnosis of major depression, drug therapy is often recommended. Tricyclic antidepressants, such as nortriptyline (Pamelor) and desipramine (Norpramin), were often prescribed in the past, but they're rarely used anymore because they may inhibit acetylcholine transmission along with causing other side effects.

The most commonly prescribed antidepressants are called selective serotonin reuptake inhibitors (SSRIs). These have proved to be effective in people with Alzheimer's while causing relatively few side effects. SSRIs act primarily by blocking serotonin receptors in the brain, yet leaving acetylcholine receptors undisturbed.

Common side effects of certain SSRIs are anxiety and agitation, and so they should be used with caution in people who already exhibit these symptoms. Other side effects include insomnia, tremor, nausea, diarrhea, headache, decreased appetite, dizziness, sweating and dry mouth. These side effects may go away on their own. Side effects may also be minimized by starting the medications at a low dose then gradually increasing to a standard dose over a period of one or two weeks.

Commonly prescribed antidepressants include:
- Citalopram (Celexa)
- Paroxetine (Paxil)
- Sertraline (Zoloft)
- Fluoxetine (Prozac)

A good perspective

The distinction between an incurable disease and an untreatable one should be noted as you contemplate the treatment options for Alzheimer's disease. It's true that, despite all the recent advances, Alzheimer's is still incurable. But it's also a treatable disease through the use of medications and personal care. Even as the symptoms of Alzheimer's progressively worsen, therapies to improve cognition, stabilize emotions and ease challenging behaviors can greatly enhance the quality of life for people with Alzheimer's and for their caregivers. A personal focus remains the strongest weapon against this unrelenting disease.

Part 3

Non-Alzheimer's forms of dementia

The following chapters focus on types of dementia that are less common than Alzheimer's but are just as devastating to those who experience them. A better understanding of these lesser known dementias may help unlock some of the mysteries surrounding all neurodegenerative disorders, including Alzheimer's.

Chapter 7

Frontotemporal dementia

Frontotemporal dementia (FTD) refers to a diverse group of neurodegenerative disorders that affect primarily the frontal and temporal lobes of your brain. See the illustration on page 26 for the location of the frontal and temporal lobes. These areas are generally associated with personality and behavior.

Neuronal damage caused by FTD often results in the impairment of "executive" skills. These are skills that allow you to function effectively in society and to interact with others, including decision making, problem solving and using good judgment. Also affected are skilled movement, language comprehension and the observance of social norms. Memory loss — one of the earliest symptoms of Alzheimer's disease — is also present but usually develops much later in the disease process.

Frontotemporal dementia tends to occur at a younger age than does Alzheimer's disease, generally between the ages of 40 and 70. Research on the incidence of FTD — how often it occurs — is still in its early stages, but study range from about 2 percent to 10 percent of all dementia cases.

The disease seems to affect men and women equally, and appears to run in the family — between 20 percent and 50 percent of people who have FTD also have a family history of some type of dementia (not only FTD). After diagnosis, the course of the disease is variable and may run anywhere from two to 10 years before resulting in death.

People with FTD, Alzheimer's or other types of dementia face similar challenges in terms of available treatment and the need for care. However, the behavioral and linguistic symptoms associated with FTD, and the earlier age of onset, present different concerns and approaches to managing the disease.

Types of frontotemporal dementia

Identifying precisely which diseases fall under the umbrella term *frontotemporal dementia* presents a particular challenge to scientists. Even when it's clear that FTD is present, the signs and symptoms of the disease may vary greatly from one individual to the next. Scientists have classified several distinct FTD subtypes based on these symptomatic differences. The symptoms are described below:

Behavioral changes. Within the general designation of FTD, there is also a subtype known as frontotemporal dementia. It is marked by extreme changes in behavior and personality. These include increasingly inappropriate actions, euphoria, lack of judgment and inhibition, apathy, repetitive compulsive behavior, and a decline in personal hygiene. The individual also demonstrates a lack of insight or awareness regarding these changes.

Speech and language comprehension. Other subtypes of frontotemporal dementia are marked by the impairment or loss of speech and linguistic capabilities (apraxia of speech and aphasia). Two subtypes of FTD produce apraxia: primary progressive aphasia, sometimes referred to as progressive nonfluent aphasia, and semantic dementia, otherwise known as progressive fluent aphasia.

Primary progressive aphasia (PPA) is characterized by difficulties in conveying meaningful sentences and finding the right words for objects, incorrect use of basic grammar, impaired comprehension, and difficulty with spelling. This subtype, which typically has an earlier onset than do other forms of FTD, may progress to include behavior and personality changes. Often people with PPA continue to function normally and are able to perform daily activi-

---

Note about FTD terminology

Dementia experts are striving to better define this group of illnesses that has a major impact on the frontal and temporal lobes of the brain. Until precise criteria are established, many aspects of FTD are subject to a particular expert's interpretation. This may be confusing, particularly when it comes to terminology. For example, frontotemporal dementia is also known as frontotemporal lobar degeneration, Pick's disease (after Arnold Pick, the doctor who first described FTD) and Pick complex.

To complicate matters, the term *frontotemporal dementia* can refer to the group of diseases as a whole and to a specific subtype of this group that primarily affects behavior. As medical experts become better acquainted with the complexities of FTD, the group and its various subtypes will become easier to describe and the terminology more standardized.

---

ties despite their language difficulties, which may result in not being able to speak at all (mutism).

Semantic dementia is characterized by spontaneous speech that's grammatically correct but bears no relevance to the conversation at hand. People with semantic dementia usually retain the ability to read and write, but they may lose the ability to recognize familiar objects or faces. As the disease progresses, behavioral changes and additional language difficulties may develop.

Movement disorders. Corticobasal degeneration (CBD) is a neurodegenerative disease that affects the frontal lobes but reveals itself primarily as a movement disorder. CBD is characterized by signs and symptoms similar to those found in Parkinson's disease (referred to as parkinsonian symptoms), such as poor coordination, rigidity, impaired balance, tremor and muscle spasms. Some people with CBD also experience alien hand syndrome, in which they can't control movement in one hand. Or they lose the ability to carry out purposeful movements, such as getting dressed or combing hair. Simple calculations, such as adding or subtracting, also may become difficult to perform. If cognitive changes do occur, they don't appear until later in the course of the disease.

Sample case of semantic dementia

After two years of persistent struggle to find words for things he wanted to say, a 53-year-old man decided to seek help from his doctor. He and his wife felt that all of his other intellectual functions were intact, including memory, language comprehension and visuospatial perception. His personality remained unchanged. His wife even noted his continued ability to tinker in the workshop and fix small engines — a task requiring considerable skill and patience.

The man was fully aware of his language difficulties and expressed significant frustration, even making self-deprecating remarks about the problem. A mental status examination showed some difficulty with abstract thinking, general knowledge awareness, construction tasks and verbal recall. Though he couldn't remember the specific words for various items on a naming test, he could describe details about each. He also had trouble understanding spoken words such as *pyramid* and *compass*. A magnetic resonance image (MRI) of his brain showed prominent shrinkage in the left temporal lobe, while the hippocampus appeared relatively preserved. These factors are fairly typical of someone with semantic dementia.

Another type of FTD that features difficulty with movement is known as frontotemporal dementia with motor neuron disease (FTD/MND). In this type of FTD, a person experiences signs and symptoms characteristic of amyotrophic lateral sclerosis (ALS, or Lou Gehrig's disease) — weakness, muscle shrinkage and muscle spasms, and swallowing difficulties — accompanied by what's generally recognized as typical symptoms of FTD. Sometimes the ALS-type symptoms develop first and are followed by symptoms of FTD, or vice versa.

People with frontotemporal dementia with parkinsonism-17 (FTDP-17), a hereditary form of FTD, have both parkinsonian symptoms and FTD symptoms.

What goes on inside the brain

Doctors can now examine the overall shape and structure of a living brain, as well as evaluate the brain's activity while performing certain tasks, with advanced imaging technology such as magnetic resonance imaging (MRI) and positron emission tomography (PET). This technology is described in Chapter 3.

Using these scans, a doctor can identify any shrinkage (atrophy) of the frontal and temporal lobes of the brain — a characteristic development of FTD — and any decreased activity in these lobes. Often specific areas where atrophy has occurred can be associated with the signs and symptoms of a FTD subtype. For example, the subtype frontotemporal dementia is marked by atrophy of both frontal lobes, while semantic dementia is often related to a degeneration of the left temporal lobe. For an example of a MRI showing frontotemporal dementia, see pages 60-61 of the Visual Guide.

Because of the difficulty of obtaining brain cell samples, a definitive examination of the brain usually must wait until an autopsy. With an opportunity to study and compare the brain tissue of people who exhibited the signs and symptoms of FTD during life, scientists have concluded that frontotemporal dementia typically has the following characteristics:

- Loss of neurons in the frontal and temporal regions
- Overgrowth of neuronal support cells (a condition known as gliosis), which forms a type of scar tissue in the brain
- Formation of tiny holes on the brain's surface in a process known as microvacuolation (mi-kro-vak-u-o-LA-shun)

About 25 percent of all cases of FTD include the presence of Pick bodies — abnormal protein-filled structures that develop within cells. Increasingly the term *Pick's disease* is being reserved only for the cases that feature these abnormal structures.

A physician also can evaluate brain tissue for the status of tau, a protein that's normally present in brain cells. Tau helps to support the cellular structure. But in a number of dementias — including Alzheimer's disease and various forms of FTD — tau is present in abnormal form or quantity, leading to a buildup of twisted strands of protein (neurofibrillary tangles) within the cells. These tangles

The genetics of FTD

From a genetic perspective, frontotemporal dementia can be seen as sporadic or familial. Many cases of FTD are sporadic, meaning there's no family history of FTD or other dementia. But in up to half the FTD cases, this form of dementia or another dementia runs in the family.

Some familial forms of frontotemporal dementia have been linked to specific genetic abnormalities (mutations). FTDP-17 is a hereditary form caused by mutations of the tau gene located on chromosome 17. FTDP-17 is inherited in an autosomal dominant pattern, which means that the child of a parent with FTDP-17 has a 50 percent chance of inheriting the disease. Currently, about 80 families worldwide have this form of FTD, representing a small percentage of all frontotemporal cases. In addition, scientists have discovered genetic links to different forms of FTD on chromosomes 3 and 9.

FTDP-17 is the only form of frontotemporal dementia for which there is genetic testing. A detailed family history, taken by a genetic counselor, helps to determine the level of risk. The genetic counselor can also help determine the risk for relatives of the person with FTD, sort through the possible outcomes, make necessary plans and identify helpful resources.

disrupt normal neuron activity and result in the death of neurons. Dementias that show tau abnormalities are sometimes called tauopathies. (For more detail on neurofibrillary tangles, see Chapter 5 and page 59 of the Visual Guide.)

Some forms of FTD have no tau abnormalities but instead have abnormalities related to the protein ubiquitin (u-BIK-wi-tin). These abnormalities are typically found in the frontal and temporal lobes, such as in FTD/MND. Other forms of FTD have both tau and ubiquitin abnormalities.

Sometimes dementias have no distinguishing characteristics except for the loss of neurons, accompanied by gliosis and microvacuolation. Doctors refer to these dementias as "lacking distinctive histology," meaning dementia with no distinctive features.

Signs and symptoms

Many combinations of signs and symptoms exist within the spectrum of frontotemporal dementia. At the same time, there are enough common characteristics among the subtypes to allow doctors to create a general description of FTD. These commonalities are helpful in diagnosis and in planning appropriate treatment.

As with other types of dementia, the nature and progression of FTD in each individual are slightly different. Not everyone experiences all of the signs and symptoms in the same way or at the same time. People with one subtype or another of FTD experience some signs and symptoms more markedly than others.

In all forms of frontotemporal dementia, changes usually occur gradually, although forms such as FTDP-17 and FTD/MND progress more rapidly than the others do. Generally, in all subtypes of FTD, behavioral and emotional changes occur before the cognitive skills decline. Memory and visuospatial orientation may be preserved for a relatively long time after diagnosis.

Below is a list of some of the general signs and symptoms of FTD, adapted in part from the Association for Frontotemporal Dementias. For more information on FTD and its subtypes, you can visit the association's Web site at *www.ftd-picks.org*.

Emotions
Emotional changes occur early in the course of frontotemporal dementia and typically include:
- Apathy toward people, surroundings and events
- Loss of emotional warmth, sympathy and empathy toward others, including loved ones
- Abrupt mood changes
- A state of exaggerated high spirits and enthusiasm (euphoria)

Behaviors
Changes in a person's social behavior and interpersonal skills are common, early signs of frontotemporal dementia. These changes gradually worsen over time and can be especially difficult to handle for family and friends. Behavioral changes may include:

Sample case of FTD

At the age of 63, a woman began experiencing gradually progressive paranoia and delusions of infidelity. Her husband noticed she wasn't paying as much attention to household chores and that she had become more socially withdrawn. She denied having any problems. She had no memory difficulty and continued to manage the household finances and to drive a car with little trouble.

Eventually, the paranoia led her to purchase a firearm, which she carried in her purse, despite the protests of her husband. One night, while she was sleeping, he took the firearm from her purse, but she purchased a replacement the next day.

Testing revealed some impairment in problem solving and intellectual flexibility, but her general intelligence, memory and visuospatial skills were normal. An MRI scan of her brain showed shrinkage of the frontal lobes.

Over the next three years, her delusions continued. She became increasingly apathetic and also developed urinary incontinence. Her case represents several characteristics typical of frontotemporal dementia.

- Loss of social skills — a decline in tactfulness and manners
- Loss of personal awareness — a decline in hygiene, for example, forgetting to bathe and change clothes
- Oral fixation — obsession with certain foods or inedible objects, overeating, excessive drinking and smoking
- Repetitive behavior — reading the same newspaper over and over, hand rubbing and clapping, humming the same tune repeatedly
- Hypersexual behavior — loss of inhibition, explicit sexual comments, obsession with pornography
- Impulsivity — impulsive buying or shoplifting, grabbing food before it's served or off someone else's plate
- Hyperactivity — agitation, pacing, vocal outbursts, aggression

Language

In certain frontotemporal subtypes, such as primary progressive aphasia and semantic dementia, problems with language and communication tend to be the primary signs and symptoms. But a decline in language skills can occur with any subtype of FTD. Language problems may include:

- Not speaking as much or reduced volume of speech (a form of aphasia)
- Difficulty speaking because of muscle weakness or incoordination (dysarthria)
- Inability to speak grammatically due to poor sentence construction and problems with tense and number (agrammatism)
- Decreased reading and writing comprehension
- Repeating the words and phrases of others (echolalia) or of one's own speech (perseveration)
- Gradual loss of all speech (mutism)

Cognition

In frontotemporal dementia, the cognitive skills that tend to decline first are the "executive" skills — decision making, problem solving, judgment, planning and adapting to change. Cognitive skills such as recent memory and visuospatial orientation may not decline until much later in the disease process. Common cognitive symptoms of FTD include:

- Difficulty focusing on a task, becoming easily distracted
- Mental inflexibility, becoming stuck in familiar patterns and having difficulty adapting to new circumstances
- Having difficulty in planning daily chores, errands and appointments and in coordinating a schedule
- Poor financial judgment

Neurological signs and symptoms

In frontotemporal subtypes such as corticobasal degeneration, FTD/MND and FTDP-17, movement disorders may occur earlier than other symptoms do. But movement-related symptoms also occur with the other subtypes. Some of the more common signs and symptoms are similar to those found in Parkinson's disease:

- Decreased facial expression
- Slowed movements
- Rigidity
- Postural instability

People with corticobasal degeneration may also experience:

- Difficulty with eye movements
- Lack of normal muscle tone
- Involuntary hand movement (alien hand syndrome)

People with FTD/MND may also experience signs and symptoms similar to those seen in amyotrophic lateral sclerosis (ALS):

- Muscle weakness
- Muscle atrophy
- Muscle spasms
- Swallowing difficulties and choking

Psychiatric symptoms

People with frontotemporal dementia may experience depression, delusions or hallucinations. The euphoria sometimes seen in people with FTD may be mistaken for mania, which is an uncontrollable, sometimes violent behavior characterized by excessive excitement and hyperactivity. It's not uncommon for a person with FTD who shows early psychiatric symptoms to be diagnosed initially with mental illness rather than dementia.

Diagnosis

The process of diagnosing frontotemporal dementia is not unlike that of diagnosing Alzheimer's disease. No single test can identify FTD, so the physician attempts to identify certain characteristic features while excluding other possible causes for the symptoms that are present. As mentioned before, because FTD affects behavior and personality, it initially may be mistaken for a mental illness, and the person may be referred to a psychiatrist.

Diagnosis of frontotemporal dementia involves the following:

- Medical evaluation of signs and symptoms and recording of a detailed medical history

How is frontotemporal dementia different from Alzheimer's?

	FTD	Alzheimer's
Age at which condition usually starts	Between ages 40 and 70	Rarely before age 65
Areas of the brain initially affected	The frontal and temporal lobes, which control personality and speech	The hippocampus, a brain structure important to memory skills; later spreads throughout brain
Progression	In early stages, personality and behavior changes; memory skills may not be lost until later stages	In early stages, increasing and persistent forgetfulness; later stages produce personality and behavior problems

- Neurological exam, which involves testing awareness and responsiveness, vital signs, reflexes, sensory responses, coordination and gait (how you walk)
- Neuropsychological testing to assess memory, ability to reason and judge, problem-solving skills, language skills, and visuospatial orientation
- Brain-imaging techniques, such as magnetic resonance imaging (MRI) and computerized tomography (CT), to check for shrinkage of the frontal and temporal lobes, and positron emission tomography (PET) and single-photon emission computerized tomography (SPECT) to evaluate brain activity

Because many questions about frontotemporal dementia remain unanswered and much is being learned from new studies, an initial diagnosis of FTD may be changed slightly at a later date. Your doctor may change the diagnosis if new signs and symptoms develop that point to a different subtype of FTD or if the criteria for diagnosis are changed. In addition, a diagnosis that's reported after an autopsy may differ from the initial diagnosis due to the presence of certain cellular characteristics or structures, such as Pick bodies, which can be identified only through the examination of brain tissue. In this example, the initial diagnosis of FTD may be changed to one of Pick's disease specifically .

Sometimes the lack of response to a particular therapy may help distinguish between disorders that share similar signs and symptoms. For example, the movement disturbances of corticobasal degeneration are sometimes confused with Parkinson's disease. If a person with parkinsonian symptoms doesn't respond to carbidopa-levodopa therapy, a medication frequently used to treat Parkinson's, this may indicate that he or she doesn't have Parkinson's and in fact has corticobasal degeneration. Other signs and symptoms, such as alien hand syndrome, may help to confirm this diagnosis.

Going through the diagnostic process can be frustrating and usually requires a generous amount of patience. But working with an experienced health professional can help determine what's causing the signs and symptoms and lead to appropriate forms of treatment and disease management.

For more detailed information on what's involved in making a diagnosis, see Chapter 3.

Treatment

There's no cure for frontotemporal dementia and no effective way to slow its progression. Treatment relies on managing the symptoms and on maintaining or improving quality of life. Some of the therapies that doctors prescribe include:

Selective serotonin reuptake inhibitors (SSRIs). People with frontotemporal dementia have a decreased level of serotonin in the brain. Serotonin is a neurotransmitter that influences mood and behavior. Doctors have found SSRIs — drugs that typically increase levels of serotonin and are administered to alleviate depression — to be of benefit for some people with FTD. SSRIs may improve signs and symptoms such as lack of inhibition, apathy, overeating and compulsive behavior.

Antipsychotics. Antipsychotics, which can block the effects of dopamine — a neurotransmitter associated with psychosis — may be of value in managing aggressive and hypersexual behavior that may develop with dementia.

Tranquilizers. If agitation or other hyperactive behaviors become problematic, small doses of tranquilizers such as trazodone may be beneficial.

Speech therapy. Speech therapy can help someone with primary progressive aphasia adjust to language difficulties and learn alternate ways to communicate.

Nutritional support. A person with FTD/MND who is having difficulty swallowing may benefit from consulting a dietitian. A dietitian can recommend foods that are nutritious but easy to swallow. As the disease progresses and eating difficulties increase, a feeding tube inserted into the stomach may be considered.

Behavioral interventions. Medications can be helpful for treating the symptoms of dementia, but they have their limitations. A caregiver's support and intervention often become necessary to provide the person with the best possible care. For example, dietary restrictions may be necessary to prevent excessive weight gain. Predictable routines and supportive guidance can be calming, while distraction and the redirection of attention can help avoid potentially difficult situations caused by aggressive behavior. For more on working with challenging behaviors, including practical tips and concrete examples, turn to the Action Guide for Caregivers on pages 278-287.

Unfortunately, acetylcholinesterase inhibitors, a group of medications commonly used to treat the early stages of Alzheimer's disease, appear to have no effect on people with frontotemporal dementia. That's why it's important to seek an early diagnosis that distinguishes FTD from Alzheimer's.

Caring for someone with frontotemporal dementia is challenging and stressful because of the extreme personality changes and behavioral problems that frequently develop. If you're a caregiver, it's vital that you seek assistance from local resources. This can come in the form of other family members and friends, support groups for caregivers, or respite care provided by adult care centers or intermittent home health care. This allows short periods of time for you to run errands or simply take a break. The Action Guide for Caregivers has more information and tips on becoming a caregiver and finding support.

Moving ahead

As scientists achieve a better understanding of the basic mechanisms of frontotemporal dementia and all of its variants, the chances of finding effective treatments increase. One thing experts are learning is that a cross-disciplinary approach — drawing on lessons learned from the clinical, pathological and genetic perspectives of the disease — is likely to be the most successful approach to FTD and other dementias. By combining knowledge from all of these areas, experts can better define the disease and create diagnostic standards. In addition, knowledge of other types of dementia may contribute to the development of new and more effective diagnostic techniques and treatments for FTD.

Chapter 8

Dementia with Lewy bodies

C hapter 1 identifies the abnormal buildup of certain proteins in the brain as a characteristic feature of many types of dementia. For example, plaques formed from the snipped fragments of amyloid precursor protein are a defining characteristic of Alzheimer's disease. The dementia type described in this chapter features distinctive structures called Lewy bodies — microscopic deposits of alpha-synuclein protein — found in deteriorating nerve cells. The existence of this protein buildup often cannot be confirmed until an autopsy is performed. While the person is alive, diagnosis and treatment are based on a careful examination and monitoring of signs and symptoms.

Overview

Dementia with Lewy bodies (DLB), with or without the presence of Alzheimer's disease, affects roughly 10 percent to 20 percent of people with dementia, making it one of the most common types of dementia. DLB becomes more common with age and affects men slightly more often than women. A few familial cases of DLB suggest that certain genes may be involved but so far, genes linked directly to the disorder have not been identified.

Alpha-synuclein protein normally is abundant in the brain, although its exact function is unknown. With abnormal function, deposits of alpha-synuclein build up within neurons to form Lewy bodies. The Lewy bodies become widespread (diffuse) throughout the brain as DLB progresses. In addition to the cognitive decline that characterizes most dementias, people with DLB usually have visual hallucinations and signs and symptoms similar to Parkinson's disease (parkinsonian symptoms), such as rigid muscles and slowed movement. These signs and symptoms fluctuate, especially in early stages of the disease.

Short history of Lewy bodies

Lewy bodies are named after German scientist Frederic H. Lewy, who first described the deposits in the brainstems of people with Parkinson's disease. After Lewy's 1913 discovery, Lewy bodies were considered a sure sign of Parkinson's. But in the 1980s, when new diagnostic techniques made the detection of the abnormal structures easier, scientists observed the widespread nature of Lewy bodies in the brains of certain individuals displaying signs and symptoms of both dementia and Parkinson's. This opened up the possibility of a new dementia type — called Lewy body disease, Lewy body dementia or senile dementia of the Lewy type.

A problem facing scientists' attempts to categorize their findings is the overlapping symptoms of Alzheimer's disease, Parkinson's disease and dementia with Lewy bodies. Lewy bodies may be present in all three disorders, although they're more widespread in DLB. Some researchers contend that DLB overlaps with Alzheimer's, while others believe the same disease mechanism underlies DLB and Parkinson's with dementia.

Research and debate regarding DLB are ongoing, but in 1996 scientists agreed on a standardized name in use today — dementia with Lewy bodies — and on specific criteria for its diagnosis. Currently, DLB is viewed as a separate disorder from Alzheimer's and Parkinson's, although this dementia type may coexist with either one.

Because the signs and symptoms of DLB are similar to those of other dementia types, particularly Alzheimer's disease, obtaining an accurate diagnosis is important. Some medications commonly used to treat psychiatric or parkinsonian symptoms may actually worsen the Lewy-body-related hallucinations and delusions.

Signs and symptoms

The changes caused by dementia with Lewy bodies can vary substantially from person to person, as can the timing of the appearance of signs and symptoms. This makes it difficult for physicians to predict how the disease will progress. Still, scientists have identified characteristic patterns that define the disease. Common signs and symptoms can be grouped into the following categories.

Cognitive impairment

The type of intellectual decline characteristic of dementia with Lewy bodies is marked by forgetfulness, attention deficit and difficulty following a single train of thought. The person appears disoriented and confused and often misidentifies people, including loved ones. He or she may have problems with depth perception and spatial orientation. Apathy and slowness of thought also may be present. All of these problems progressively worsen.

A distinctive feature of DLB is the very noticeable fluctuations in alertness and in the ability to perform complex cognitive tasks and solve problems, especially early in the disease process. Confusion, disorientation, reduced attention or even severe sleepiness may last for minutes, hours or days, interspersed with periods of normal or near-normal functioning.

Psychiatric symptoms

People with DLB often have visual hallucinations involving vivid, colorful images of people and animals — although no sounds usually accompany the images. The hallucinations can range from funny to very frightening to the people having them. Some attempt to talk to or shoo away these perceived images, and they become upset if someone tries to convince them that what they see isn't real. Others are aware that their perceptions are false and manage to carry on as normal. Hallucinations may occur during the day, but they're more often experienced at night.

Delusions, which are false beliefs, also are common with DLB. People may become paranoid and susceptible to conspiracy theories, believing, for example, that someone is stealing from them or that an impostor has replaced a spouse.

Visual illusions may occur, in which the person believes a real object is something other than what it is, such as imagining an ornate lamppost to be an animal or a person.

As with other types of dementia, depression and anxiety also commonly occur. However, these conditions may improve with treatment.

Why dementia with Lewy bodies causes these psychiatric symptoms is uncertain, but it may be associated with the disruption of certain neurotransmitters in the brain, such as dopamine, acetylcholine and serotonin. Sleep disorders that typically accompany DLB also may play a role.

Motor symptoms

At some point during the course of the illness, many people with DLB develop parkinsonian signs and symptoms. These signs and symptoms, which primarily affect muscle function, may include:

- Slowed movements
- Stooped or leaning posture
- Difficulty manipulating facial muscles, resulting in frequent blank expressions
- Tendency to drool
- Muscle stiffness and rigidity
- Balance problems
- Shuffling walk (gait)
- Difficulty with refined motor skills — for example, handwriting or buttoning a shirt
- Tremor or shaking (not as common as in Parkinson's disease)

Although all of these cognitive, psychiatric and motor symptoms are common with DLB, some people may never experience them during the illness. When they don't occur, it may be easy to mistake DLB for another type of dementia.

Sleep disorders

Common to illnesses that involve a buildup of alpha-synuclein protein — such as DLB, Parkinson's disease and multiple system atrophy — are sleep disorders, particularly a condition known as rapid eye movement sleep behavior disorder, also known as RBD.

RBD is a sleep disorder in which people appear to act out their dreams — often involving being chased or attacked. Those with RBD may yell, scream, punch, kick or otherwise try to defend themselves from an attacker in their dreams. If awakened, their vivid dream descriptions usually match the intensity of their actions, which can be dangerous to the dreamer as well as to a spouse or partner sleeping in the same bed. RBD tends to precede other symptoms of dementia with Lewy bodies by several years.

Other sleep disorders associated with this dementia include insomnia, sleep apnea and restless legs syndrome. Perhaps as a result of sleep disorders, a person with DLB may experience drowsiness, nodding off periodically during the day.

Sleep disorders can be treated separately from DLB. Treatment may help improve alertness and lessen the fluctuating periods of confusion or disorientation. In some cases, treating the sleep disorders decreases or eliminates visual hallucinations.

Autonomic dysfunction

In DLB, the autonomic nervous system — which controls involuntary muscle movements such as blood vessel, bladder and bowel contractions— is frequently impaired. This results in signs and symptoms such as:

- Lightheadedness or dizziness upon standing, a result of a dramatic drop in blood pressure (orthostatic hypotension)
- Fainting
- Frequent falls, resulting from dizziness or fainting
- Impotence
- Urinary incontinence
- Constipation

Diagnosis

Doctors must diagnose dementia with Lewy bodies on the basis of the signs and symptoms described above. No biological test is available that positively identifies DLB — a definitive diagnosis is possible only at autopsy. At that time, a pathologist examines the brain tissue for Lewy bodies in the brainstem, limbic system and regions of the cerebral cortex.

Cognitive decline and two of the following features *must* be present for a physician to be fairly certain that the signs and symptoms represent DLB (known as a "probable" diagnosis).

- Noticeable fluctuations in cognition (memory, reason, judgment) with varying levels of alertness
- Recurrent visual hallucinations
- Spontaneous parkinsonian symptoms (which means there's no evidence these symptoms are caused by taking medications or by any other identifiable factor)

If at least one feature in this bulleted list is present, along with cognitive decline, the physician may consider the possibility of DLB (known as a "possible" diagnosis).

Although additional signs and symptoms of DLB aren't essential to a diagnosis, knowledge of them may give the doctor a more complete picture of the condition. This information may come from family and friends willing to share their observations.

Tests to help with a diagnosis of DLB are similar to those in use for other dementias. (See Chapter 3 for more about tests used in diagnosing dementia.) People with DLB often have greater problems with attention, concentration and visuospatial skills, but less trouble with naming objects and verbal memory. Brain scans reveal that atrophy of the hippocampus area frequently is less severe in DLB than in Alzheimer's or vascular cognitive impairment.

Dementia with Lewy bodies and Alzheimer's

Dementia with Lewy bodies causes many of the same signs and symptoms of cognitive decline that Alzheimer's disease does. In fact, DLB is often mistaken for Alzheimer's. Autopsies reveal that the brain tissue of most people with DLB also contains the characteristic features of Alzheimer's, such as amyloid plaques and neu-rofibrillary tangles, in addition to Lewy bodies. Doctors may refer to this combination as "DLB coexisting with Alzheimer's disease."

Scientists note that people with DLB who have few tangles tend to show primarily the symptoms of DLB, while those with many tangles exhibit symptoms closer to those of Alzheimer's.

On the other hand, brain tissue of some people with Alzheimer's will contain Lewy bodies, even though no symptoms of DLB are apparent. This raises the question, still unanswered, of whether DLB and Alzheimer's are related in some way.

Dementia with Lewy bodies and Parkinson's

Lewy bodies often appear within the brainstems of people with Parkinson's disease. In fact, dementia can occur in conjunction with Parkinson's — usually referred to as Parkinson's disease with dementia, or PDD. This form of Parkinson's is very similar to DLB, differing only in the timing of the occurrence of symptoms. If parkinsonian symptoms occur more than a year before dementia symptoms begin, doctors generally consider this to be PDD rather than DLB.

Scientists debate whether the disease mechanisms that underlie DLB and PDD are the same or if they're two distinct disorders. Most evidence suggests that DLB and PDD are variants of the same disease. With so many uncertainties and possible connections to other conditions, a diagnosis of DLB is difficult. And the diagnosis may change during the course of the illness or even after death.

Treatment

Because the underlying cause of dementia with Lewy bodies is still unknown, treatment is aimed at lessening the impact of symptoms on quality of life. This typically involves a combination of caregiving, nondrug interventions and possibly medications. People with DLB and their caregivers can play important roles in therapy by identifying symptoms that they feel need the most attention, even if those symptoms and needs change over time.

Caregiving

As with all forms of dementia, caregiving is one of the most important and humane components of DLB therapy. Caregiving can provide physical, emotional and spiritual support in challenging times. Most of all, caregiving can ensure that the doctor's recommendations for treatment are carried out and improve quality of life.

Sample case of dementia with Lewy body

Dr. X is a physician who developed dementia with Lewy bodies in his early 70s. Although no two cases are exactly alike, Dr. X experienced what could be considered the classic signs and symptoms of DLB.

At age 72, Dr. X began to experience difficulties in dictating notes, counseling patients and writing prescriptions. This caused him to retire from his profession the following year. At about the same time, he started having trouble expressing himself and frequently lost his train of thought during conversations. He would forget recent events, make incorrect turns while driving and miscalculate numbers in his head. His thinking slowed, as did his normal walking pace. His wife noticed that some hours or days were far better than others. The doctor himself, a keen observer of his symptoms, noticed he was developing dressing apraxia — trouble putting on his clothes correctly.

Of some concern was the fact that both his sister and maternal uncle had developed dementia in their late 60s. Dr. X also had a history of depression, for which medical therapy was only moderately effective. About 10 years earlier, he had developed impotence and more recently felt lightheaded upon standing, nearly fainting on several occasions. Testing revealed that Dr. X had low blood pressure.

His wife noted that, beginning nine years earlier, he would often yell, curse and vigorously shake his legs while sleeping, as if he were "acting out his dreams." When she woke him, he

Because of the rigorous demands, it's essential for caregivers to obtain education and support — from doctors, community health centers, dementia support groups or other sources of assistance. For more information, see the Action Guide for Caregivers on pages 218-329. For information about DLB, visit the Lewy Body Dementia Association's Web site at *www.lewybodydementia.org.*

described being chased by people or animals. Further testing revealed a form of sleep apnea for which his doctor prescribed therapy that improved his alertness, concentration and mood.

His doctor prescribed a cholinesterase inhibitor traditionally used for Alzheimer's, which improved some cognitive symptoms. Therapy normally intended for Parkinson's was then added, resulting in improvement of his motor symptoms.

Some months later, Dr. X left on a tropical vacation with his wife. Shortly after checking into the hotel, he experienced visual hallucinations and delusions. At the local emergency room, his wife requested that treatment be given, but she specifically instructed the medical staff not to give haloperidol, a conventional antipsychotic frequently used for hallucinations. The staff did so nonetheless, as Dr. X's symptoms were worsening. Hours later, Dr. X developed extreme sleepiness and muscle stiffness.

Transferred to another hospital, Dr. X was started on a low dosage of quetiapine, a newer antipsychotic that has fewer adverse effects on people with DLB. Eventually, his mental state improved significantly, although the muscle stiffness persisted.

For two years, Dr. X's symptoms remained fairly stable. Ever the doctor, he remarked at one point, "I clearly meet criteria for dementia, but my psychosis and depression have remained in check. My orthostatism (lightheadedness from low blood pressure) is my most troubling issue right now."

Nondrug treatment

Much can be done to improve the quality of life of someone with DLB without using medication. This is where education and awareness of others' experience often play a vital role. These resources may be adapted to suit your specific situation.

For example, Dr. X from the case study in this chapter described lightheadedness as an ongoing concern in treating DLB. Low blood pressure leading to orthostatic hypotension can be managed in several ways — by increasing dietary salt intake, by using thigh-high compression stockings or elastic abdominal support garments, and by elevating the head of the bed about 30 degrees.

To decrease risk of injury from nighttime concerns such as rapid eye movement sleep behavior disorder (RBD), consider moving lamps and nightstands away from the bed and placing padding or cushions on the floor beside the bed, in case of a fall. If a bed partner is at risk, sleeping in separate beds should be considered.

In addition, the doctor may request a careful sleep history or monitor sleep patterns to determine if sleep apnea is present. This can be done by using a machine that delivers air pressure through a mask placed over the nose (continuous positive airway pressure therapy, or CPAP). Rearranging the dosing periods of drugs that may cause insomnia, such as cholinesterase inhibitors, also may help improve sleep.

Medications

Medications are often necessary to help treat the cognitive, psychiatric and parkinsonian symptoms of DLB. Medications intended for sleep disorders, insomnia and low blood pressure — which often are concurrent and treatable conditions — also may improve the quality of life for someone with DLB.

It's worth repeating how important it is to obtain an accurate diagnosis, ideally from a doctor experienced in treating dementia, such as a neurologist or neuropsychiatrist. That's because some common medications for treating general psychiatric and parkinsonian symptoms can actually make the DLB symptoms worse. The dosages and side effects of the various drugs must be continuously adjusted and balanced for optimal benefit.

Here are medications that may prove helpful in treating DLB:

Cholinesterase inhibitors. Both Alzheimer's disease and dementia with Lewy bodies are characterized by a sharp drop in levels of acetylcholine, a vital neurotransmitter that's important in thinking and memory skills.

Cholinesterase inhibitors were originally designed to treat the cognitive losses of Alzheimer's by inhibiting the enzyme acetylcholinesterase. This enzyme breaks down acetylcholine immediately after the neurotransmitter has done its primary job — triggering a nerve cell to send an impulse. In effect, the enzyme's action cancels out the acetylcholine's availability to trigger additional messages between nerve cells. By blocking this enzyme, cholinesterase inhibitors allow the acetylcholine to remain available and trigger more nerve impulses, thereby improving cognition.

Interestingly, cholinesterase inhibitors often appear to be more effective in treating dementia with Lewy bodies than in treating Alzheimer's. This may be because the damage to neurons may be less severe in DLB than in Alzheimer's.

In DLB, the cholinesterase inhibitors help temper the fluctuating nature of the cognitive deficits and improve problems with hallucinations, apathy, anxiety and sleep. However, these drugs may cause gastrointestinal side effects and excessive salivation, and they may also increase the risk of falls.

For more about cholinesterase inhibitors, see pages 99-101.

Antipsychotics. Conventional antipsychotic medications such as haloperidol (Haldol) — often used to treat hallucinations, delusions and agitation — can provoke severe reactions in individuals with DLB, leading to irreversible losses of certain motor skills. Some newer antipsychotics — risperidone (Risperdal), olanzapine (Zyprexa), quetiapine (Seroquel) and clozapine (Clozaril) — may cause fewer side effects while improving symptoms. But their use requires careful monitoring, as there are reports of negative reactions to these medications as well, and of slightly increased risk of death.

Caregivers and doctors should make sure that all health care providers are aware of the person's condition and that prescriptions of antipsychotics are monitored appropriately.

Anti-parkinsonian drugs. Medications commonly used to treat parkinsonian symptoms need close monitoring in people with dementia with Lewy bodies. Two examples are carbidopa-levodopa and dopamine agonists — drugs that convert to or mimic the effects of dopamine, a neurotransmitter important in muscle control and movement. Unfortunately, these drugs may also worsen psychotic symptoms and orthostatic hypotension. As a result, these medications are given at the lowest possible doses.

Antidepressants. Depression is common in people with DLB, likely because of a decline in levels of the neurotransmitter serotonin. One class of antidepressants will increase levels of active serotonin in the brain — selective serotonin reuptake inhibitors (SSRIs). These medications are usually helpful for depression and anxiety, with generally tolerable side effects. Tricyclic antidepressants aren't helpful in treating DLB, as they will reduce an already depleted reserve of the neurotransmitter acetylcholine.

Memantine. Memantine (Namenda) has modestly improved functional abilities in people with moderate to severe dementia associated with Alzheimer's. While memantine has yet to be proved effective in DLB, some physicians may recommend using it in select people.

All for one, one for all

Unraveling the enigmatic mysteries that may link dementia with Lewy bodies to Alzheimer's disease and to Parkinson's disease remains a perplexing issue for physicians and scientists. As research continues to progress in the search for more effective therapies for Alzheimer's and Parkinson's, advances in these fields may ultimately benefit people with DLB.

Chapter 9

Vascular cognitive impairment

Vascular cognitive impairment is notable among the major types of dementia — which also include Alzheimer's disease, frontotemporal dementia and dementia with Lewy bodies — because its cause is fairly well understood. When blood flow in the brain is disrupted and insufficient amounts of oxygen and nutrients reach brain cells, the result is cell damage or death. Areas of damaged or dead brain tissue, known as infarcts, remain at these locations and are not replaced by new cells. Depending on their location, these damaged areas can produce losses of cognition, personality and emotional health.

In recent years, the term *vascular cognitive impairment* (VCI) has begun to be used in place of the former term, *vascular dementia*. This name shift reflects the fact that vascular disease is capable of causing cognitive impairment in the brain without necessarily meeting the standard criteria that define dementia.

Because vascular cognitive impairment is caused by unhealthy blood vessels, factors such as high blood pressure and atherosclerosis have a major impact on a person's risk of VCI. Unlike other dementias, many aspects of which remain a mystery, preventive steps can be taken to reduce this risk and to stop further damage to the brain if the signs and symptoms of vascular cognitive impairment begin to appear.

Overview

As the central control room of your body, your brain requires a substantial supply of blood — about 20 percent of your heart's total output. Four main arteries converge at the base of your brain, from which a network of smaller and smaller blood vessels reaches deep into the brain interior. Whenever there's an interruption in your brain's blood supply, depriving cells of essential nutrients such as oxygen and glucose, these cells are rapidly damaged or die.

Stroke is a common result of blood flow disruption in the brain. Stroke occurs when a blood clot blocks an artery or when an artery leaks or ruptures, bleeding into the surrounding tissue. This disruption of blood flow — even for a few seconds — usually has a dramatic effect on your brain's function.

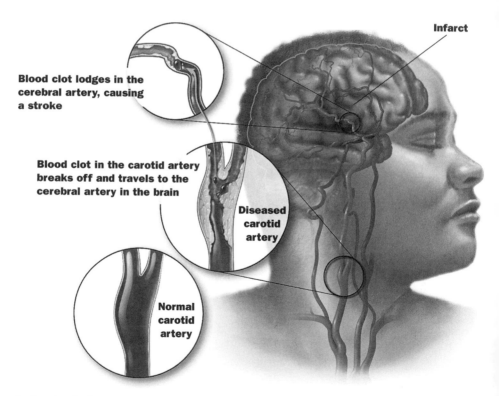

Ischemic stroke may occur when a blood clot (thrombus) forms in an area of atherosclerosis. Turbulent blood flow around deposits of plaques may trigger this clot development. This can occur in the carotid artery of the neck or in other arteries.

Most of us think of stroke as a major event that causes severe impairment of movement and speech. A major stroke such as this can permanently damage structures important to cognitive function and lead to vascular cognitive impairment.

But strokes may also occur on a smaller and "silent" level in which symptoms from a single event, if any, are minimal. However, a series of these minor strokes may damage enough brain cells to cause dementia. In addition, if the small blood vessels throughout the brain become weak and narrow due to vascular disease, a reduced blood supply may damage or destroy tissue, even if the blood vessels aren't completely blocked or ruptured.

Before recent advances in the understanding of Alzheimer's disease, doctors believed most cases of dementia had a vascular source — due to diseased arteries in the brain. Because research now suggests that Alzheimer's — the most common form of dementia — is likely a result of multiple factors, the frequency of dementia associated with vascular disease has become a matter of debate.

One problem is the difficulty of reaching even a rough estimate of the number of new cases. Because there are varying definitions of VCI and different sets of criteria for its diagnosis, it's hard to reach a consensus on prevalence. A complicating factor is that VCI and Alzheimer's disease frequently coexist, so diagnosis of one may not rule out the presence of the other.

As a result, estimates of vascular cognitive impairment range widely, from one-tenth to one-third of all dementia cases. A common opinion is that for every four or five people with Alzheimer's, there may be one with VCI. In the population as a whole, estimates of vascular cognitive impairment among adults age 65 or older range from 1 percent to 4 percent.

Mechanisms of the disease process

In the medical sense, *mechanism* refers to any combination of physical and chemical processes that cause an action or reaction to take place in the body. Scientists are studying the interconnections between several processes while trying to understand the causes of

VCI. Certain mechanisms have been identified that could cause the disorder. These include:

A series of infarcts. In this circumstance, a person experiences a series of small or large strokes, each one resulting in an infarct, or area of dead brain tissue. Even if they're all small ones, enough infarcts gradually create enough damage to cause dementia. In fact, all forms of vascular cognitive impairment were once referred to as multi-infarct dementia — reflecting conventional thinking that multiple strokes were behind the condition. But it's also true that a single, strategically located stroke (see below) can cause cognitive impairment, so the term *multi-infarct dementia* is no longer considered an accurate description of the disease.

Single strategic infarct. Sometimes a single stroke affecting a critical area of the brain — such as the thalamus or parietal lobe — can cause a sudden onset of dementia. As stated in Chapter 2, the thalamus acts as your brain's switchboard for processing information, and the parietal lobe is the part of the brain that receives sensory information and supports visuospatial abilities. Severe damage to either of these regions dramatically affects cognition.

Stroke and vascular cognitive impairment

Vascular cognitive impairment commonly occurs in people who have had a major stroke. According to some estimates, between 20 percent and 30 percent of people who've had a stroke go on to develop dementia, usually within several months of the event. One study found that having a stroke doubles a person's risk of dementia. Findings such as this support the belief that preventing stroke is a major step in preventing vascular cognitive impairment.

But that doesn't mean all strokes lead to VCI. Although stroke can cause confusion, memory loss, and difficulties with language and perception, these effects are usually at their worst immediately after the stroke and may improve gradually over time. This type of temporary cognitive impairment isn't the same thing as dementia, the signs and symptoms of which progressively become worse.

Small vessel disease. As its name implies, this disease affects the small blood vessels of the brain and is closely associated with high blood pressure. Widespread damage from blocked vessels and chronic reduction in blood flow leads to a slower, more subtle onset of dementia. Some scientists believe that a "microvascular" disease such as this may be more damaging to the brain than larger "macrovascular" strokes involving the major arteries.

Two examples of small vessel disease are Binswanger's disease, which affects the white matter deep inside the brain, and cerebral autosomal dominant arteriopathy with subcortical infarcts and leukoencephalopathy (CADASIL), a rare inherited form of VCI caused by a genetic defect on chromosome 19.

Combined Alzheimer's disease and VCI. Autopsy reports indicate that the brains of many people diagnosed with dementia show signs of both Alzheimer's disease and VCI. It appears that when the two occur together, one compounds the effects of the other, leading to a more severe form of dementia. A growing number of researchers are working on understanding the relationship between vascular cognitive impairment and Alzheimer's.

Signs and symptoms

People with vascular cognitive impairment experience many of the same signs and symptoms as do people with Alzheimer's disease or other dementias. For example, memory loss is a common complaint — although people with VCI may respond better to memory cues and reminders than may people with Alzheimer's. Other signs and symptoms include:
- Apathy
- Confusion
- Wandering or getting lost in familiar places
- Difficulty with problem solving, organizing and planning
- Walking disturbances
- Loss of bowel or bladder control
- Sudden, involuntary laughing and crying
- Hallucinations and delusions

In what may be considered a classic example of VCI — a person experiencing a series of small or large strokes — the disorder may follow a stepwise progression, with symptoms plateauing or remaining steady until the next stroke occurs, causing further damage and additional symptoms.

The types and intensities of symptoms depend on the location of the infarcts, so some cognitive functions may become impaired while others are preserved. For example, a person with VCI may have trouble following instructions but still be fairly conscious of his or her impairment. This can be frustrating for the person and increase the depression that often accompanies the disorder.

Sample case of vascular dementia

An independent 80-year-old woman living on her own experienced a stroke that, on a computerized tomography (CT) scan, appeared to affect only the occipital lobe of her brain — often known as the visual cortex. Although her symptoms improved immediately after the stroke, her son observed a noticeable decline in her cognition and physical abilities. One year after her stroke, she was able to dress and feed herself but needed help with most other activities of daily living, including bathing. She could no longer drive, pay bills or do household chores. She also became increasingly quiet and withdrawn. Although she was able to write and could name a few simple items, she was unable to read.

Another brain-imaging test, this time a magnetic resonance image (MRI), showed that the stroke had damaged not only the occipital lobe but also the hippocampus and thalamus, two structures important in memory and information processing. This helped explain the cause of her dementia. However, her doctors couldn't be sure that she had no preexisting cognitive impairment that may have contributed to her dementia or been exacerbated by her stroke.

A person in the early stages of vascular cognitive impairment may experience greater physical disability — loss of motor skills, for example — than may someone in the early stages of Alzheimer's disease. And, in general, people with Alzheimer's live longer than do those with vascular cognitive impairment, in whom heart disease and stroke are more likely to be a cause of death.

Some cases of vascular cognitive impairment, however — especially those caused by small vessel disease — may progress in similar fashion as Alzheimer's disease, with a slow but steady decline in cognitive and, eventually, physical functions.

Risk factors

As you age, your blood vessels become more prone to the accumulation of fatty deposits (plaques) containing cholesterol and other substances. When compounded by a lack of exercise and a cholesterol-heavy diet, the buildup of these plaques leads to a narrowing and hardening of your blood vessels (atherosclerosis), making it more difficult for blood to flow through them. In addition, chronic high blood pressure makes the walls of your blood vessels weak and more susceptible to rupture. Both atherosclerosis and high blood pressure can make you more susceptible to vascular diseases, including VCI, stroke and heart disease.

Other factors that put you at risk of vascular diseases include diabetes, smoking and unhealthy cholesterol levels. Managing these risk factors is important in the prevention and treatment of vascular cognitive impairment.

Risk factors for vascular disease beyond your control — but that you still should be aware of — include advancing age, male sex and African-American ethnicity. Carrying the apolipoprotein ε4 allele also is a risk factor for VCI, as it is for Alzheimer's disease (for more on this allele, see pages 92-93). But having this gene variant doesn't guarantee that you'll develop dementia, any more than lacking the variant means you won't. Because there's little benefit from knowing whether you carry the allele, doctors don't recommend testing for it.

Diagnosis

The process of diagnosing vascular cognitive impairment is similar to diagnosing other dementias, and includes a review of medical history, assessment of signs and symptoms, physical and neurological exams, neuropsychological tests to evaluate memory and cognitive function, and brain-imaging tests such as magnetic resonance imaging (MRI) and computerized tomography (CT) scans. (For more details on these tests, see Chapter 3).

Different criteria may be used for a diagnosis of vascular cognitive impairment, so an evaluation will depend on which set of criteria the doctor adheres to. In general, however, three characteristic features will indicate that the signs and symptoms are a result of vascular cognitive impairment instead of other causes:

- Onset or worsening of cognitive losses within three months of having a stroke
- Evidence of one or more strokes on brain imaging tests
- Signs and symptoms consistent with what's occurred after previous strokes, such as a nerve problem limited to a specific location (left or right side of the body) or a specific function (speech or fine-motor skill)

Distinguishing vascular cognitive impairment from Alzheimer's disease may be one of the most challenging aspects of a diagnosis. Although often there's a clear association between the occurrence of a stroke and later development of dementia, in other cases this connection isn't apparent. Symptoms of VCI can be very similar to symptoms of Alzheimer's, and without the evidence of stroke, it may be virtually impossible to deduce whether the cause of dementia is vascular. That's why brain imaging, such as CT scans and MRIs, is perhaps the most useful tool in diagnosing VCI — it often provides evidence of stroke in the absence of any external signs and symptoms. For example, infarcts show up as white, clouded regions on the CT scan on page 62.

Vascular cognitive impairment may develop as a result of infarcts so small that they're undetectable even with brain imaging. In such instances, a diagnosis of Alzheimer's will frequently be made, and VCI may not be recognized until after an examination of brain tissue during autopsy. It's also possible for a person to have both forms of dementia, so the diagnosis of one doesn't necessarily rule out the presence of the other.

In spite of these difficulties and uncertainties, it's vital to identify the presence of vascular cognitive impairment when it develops. By managing vascular risk factors such as high blood pressure and high cholesterol, you may be able to diminish the severity of this disorder. You may even lessen the impact of Alzheimer's disease, should it coexist with VCI.

Treatment and prevention

Damage to brain tissue can't be reversed — what's done is done. So the treatment of vascular cognitive impairment consists of preventing any further damage from occurring. This means avoiding further strokes by managing risk factors that are under your control, such as blood pressure and cholesterol levels. This may help to limit the severity of the disorder or delay its progression. Even in the absence of stroke, taking preventive steps can help you reduce your risk of developing VCI.

Scientists remain uncertain about the relationship between vascular risk factors and the development of Alzheimer's disease, but several studies show a positive correlation. As mentioned before, vascular cognitive impairment may increase the severity of Alzheimer's disease when both conditions are present. Therefore, the steps taken to prevent stroke may have a beneficial effect on Alzheimer's, as well.

Preventing stroke

Whether or not you've experienced a stroke, it's important to know where you stand in terms of its risk factors. Follow your doctor's advice if you need to change behaviors and lifestyle. Your doctor also may prescribe medications to help you reach those goals. Here are ways to reduce your risk of stroke and VCI:

Control high blood pressure (hypertension). One of the most important things you can do to reduce your risk of stroke is to keep your blood pressure under control. If you've already had a stroke, lowering your blood pressure can help prevent a subsequent stroke. Exercising, managing stress, maintaining a healthy weight, and limiting sodium and alcohol intake are all ways to keep hypertension in check. In addition, your doctor may prescribe medications to reduce hypertension, such as diuretics, angiotensin-converting enzyme (ACE) inhibitors and angiotensin receptor blockers.

In a study of over 6,000 older adults, the ACE inhibitor perindopril (Aceon) combined with the diuretic indapamide (Lozol), was shown to reduce the risk of dementia and severe cognitive impairment by 12 percent among people who had recurrent stroke.

Lower your cholesterol and saturated fat intake. Eating less cholesterol and fat, especially saturated fat, may reduce the buildup of fatty deposits in your arteries. Your doctor may prescribe a cholesterol-lowering medication such as a statin.

Take B vitamins. B complex vitamins — B-6, B-12 and folic acid (folate) — can work together to reduce blood levels of homocysteine. Excessive levels of this protein in your blood may increase your risk of blood vessel damage.

Don't smoke. Stopping smoking reduces your risk of stroke. Several years after stopping, a former smoker's risk of stroke is the same as that of a nonsmoker.

Control diabetes. You can manage diabetes with diet, exercise, weight control and medication. Strict control of your blood sugar may reduce the damage to your brain if you do have a stroke.

Maintain a healthy weight. Being overweight contributes to other risk factors for stroke, such as high blood pressure, cardiovascular disease and diabetes. Weight loss of as little as 10 pounds may lower your blood pressure and improve your cholesterol levels.

Exercise regularly. Aerobic exercise, which strengthens your breathing and heart rates, can also reduce your risk of stroke. This exercise can lower your blood pressure, increase your level of "good" high-density lipoprotein (HDL) cholesterol, and improve the overall health of your blood vessels and heart. It also helps you lose weight, control diabetes and reduce stress. Gradually work up to 30 minutes of activity — such as walking, jogging, swimming or bicycling — on most, if not all, days of the week.

Manage stress. Stress can cause a temporary spike in your blood pressure — a risk factor for brain hemorrhage — or long-lasting hypertension. It can also increase your blood's tendency to clot, which may elevate your risk of a blocked artery. Simplifying your life, exercising and using relaxation techniques are all approaches that you can learn to reduce stress.

Drink alcohol in moderation, if at all. Alcohol can be both a risk factor and a preventive measure for stroke. Binge drinking and heavy alcohol consumption increase your risk of high blood pressure and stroke. However, drinking small to moderate amounts of alcohol may increase your HDL cholesterol and decrease your blood's tendency to clot. Either factor may contribute to a lower risk of stroke, but this can also be achieved without drinking.

Don't use illicit drugs. Many street drugs, such as cocaine, are associated with a high risk of stroke.

A brain-healthy diet

Eating nutritious foods helps keep your arteries clog-free so they can provide your brain with a nutrient-rich supply of blood. A brain-healthy diet should include:

- Five or more daily servings of fruits and vegetables, which contain nutrients such as potassium, folate and antioxidants that may protect against stroke
- Foods rich in soluble fiber, such as oatmeal and beans
- Foods rich in calcium, a mineral that reduces stroke risk
- Soy products such as tempeh, miso, tofu and soy milk, which can reduce your "bad" low-density lipoprotein (LDL) cholesterol and raise your "good" high-density lipoprotein (HDL) cholesterol levels
- Foods rich in omega-3 fatty acids, including cold-water fish such as salmon, mackerel and tuna

Dementia medications

Several studies have found that the cholinesterase inhibitors galantamine (Razadyne, formerly known as Reminyl) and donepezil (Aricept) — both used to treat Alzheimer's disease — may be effective in treating vascular cognitive impairment. They may be especially beneficial in people with both VCI and Alzheimer's. As with Alzheimer's, these drugs may slow the progression of vascular cognitive impairment but they can't cure it.

Cholinesterase inhibitors help to increase the levels of acetylcholine, a neurotransmitter associated with memory function, by inhibiting the activity of enzymes that break up acetylcholine. People with Alzheimer's experience a dramatic drop in acetylcholine levels as the disease progresses. In vascular cognitive impairment, structures associated with acetylcholine production are susceptible to damage caused by high blood pressure, which may reduce the level of acetylcholine in the brain.

Positive steps toward prevention

One of the best ways to maintain the vital cognitive functions of memory, judgment and reason, is to prevent the development of vascular cognitive impairment. That's why it's so important to know your risk factors for stroke. Ask your doctor's advice about how best to control these factors.

As brain-imaging technology improves, doctors will be able to better identify the strokes that cause dementia, resulting in more accurate diagnosis and appropriate treatment. They may even be able to view microscopic changes in the inner brain that are not visible with current technology.

In addition, greater understanding about the complex relationship between vascular cognitive impairment and Alzheimer's disease may help doctors arrive at a consensus for diagnosis, and potentially better treatments.

Chapter 10

Other causes of dementia

In addition to the neurodegenerative and vascular disorders described in preceding chapters, there are many other conditions that can damage the brain and cause dementia. These have been grouped in a single chapter because, as dementing disorders go, they may seem relatively rare in relation to conditions such as Alzheimer's disease and vascular cognitive impairment.

However, being rare doesn't make these conditions any less worthy of attention or any less devastating for the individual contracting one of them. Furthermore, the results from a study of one of these conditions may provide valuable insight into the causes of dementia or provide the key to a new treatment that has applications for other forms of dementia.

There are, nevertheless, common features among the various and seemingly disparate conditions described in this chapter. A few are genetic, passed on from parent to child. In several examples, the dementia is secondary — a complication of a separate illness.

Although most of these causes of dementia are irreversible and treatment is based primarily on managing the symptoms, there are exceptions that may be treatable, such as normal pressure hydrocephalus. Where dementia is a complication of another illness, treatment of the underlying cause may help stop or delay the progression of cognitive loss.

Normal pressure hydrocephalus

Hydrocephalus is a condition in which the cerebrospinal fluid that surrounds and cushions the brain and fills its cavities (ventricles) doesn't drain as it should. Instead, the fluid builds up, causing an abnormal enlargement of the ventricles and increased pressure on the brain, potentially damaging the brain. It's most commonly recognized as a congenital (existing at birth) disorder.

In adults, a variation of hydrocephalus called normal pressure hydrocephalus may occur. In this variation, measurements of cerebrospinal fluid pressure fall within a normal range, but the reabsorption of fluid is defective. This causes the ventricles of the brain to enlarge, but not under high pressure. Enlargement of the ventricles compresses brain tissue and can cause cognitive impairment, difficulty with walking and loss of bladder control.

This type of hydrocephalus is most often seen in older adults and may be the result of an injury or illness, but in the majority of cases the cause is unknown. Sometimes normal pressure hydrocephalus may be treatable.

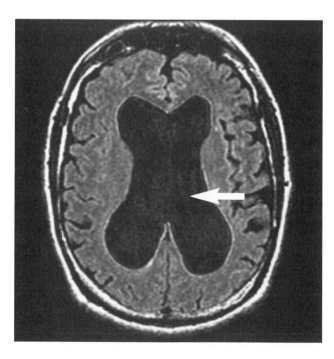

Normal pressure hydrocephalus

With this condition, cerebrospinal fluid pressure is normal, but reabsorption of the fluid is defective. Enlargement of the ventricles (see arrow) compresses brain tissue, causing cognitive impairment.

Signs and symptoms

The three hallmark characteristics of normal pressure hydrocephalus include:

Difficulty walking. Usually the first symptom to present itself
may be walking slowly with short, shuffling steps. A person with
normal pressure hydrocephalus will tend to walk with his or her
feet spread wide. Difficulty starting to move, lack of balance and
frequent falls also are common.

Urinary incontinence. Deformation of the nerve fibers that control the bladder can lead to stronger and more frequent urges to
urinate, which may cause incontinence. These signs and symptoms
usually follow the appearance of walking difficulties.

Dementia. Dementia often reveals itself in normal pressure
hydrocephalus as an overall slowness in thinking and information
processing, as well as inattention and lack of spontaneity. The signs
and symptoms may not appear to be as severe as those of disorders
described in other chapters. Unlike people with Alzheimer's disease, for example, people with normal pressure hydrocephalus usually can answer a question correctly, although it may take a bit
longer than normal to reply.

The signs and symptoms of normal pressure hydrocephalus are
common to other forms of dementia, which can sometimes lead to
misdiagnosis. However, the pattern in which they develop often is
different — from Alzheimer's in particular. A careful evaluation by
a neurologist or neurosurgeon will reveal the differences. Brain
imaging tests and a spinal tap can help rule out other possible conditions. Early diagnosis helps in that appropriate treatment can be
started for those who might benefit from it.

Treatment

Normal pressure hydrocephalus can be treated by draining excess
cerebrospinal fluid from the brain through a shunt system. To do
this, a surgeon places the end of a long, flexible tube in one of the
brain's ventricles. From the ventricle, the tube is tunneled beneath
the scalp and under the skin along the neck and chest down to the
abdomen, where the fluid is allowed to drain. This normalizes the
fluid level in the brain and may help to relieve symptoms.

Although treatment helps many people with normal pressure hydrocephalus, not everyone improves, and for some, improvement may be temporary. Not many well-designed trials have been conducted on normal pressure hydrocephalus, so it's difficult to estimate the success rate. A review of several small studies found that about 60 percent of participants with normal pressure hydrocephalus improved after the shunting procedure, but only about half of these people experienced continued improvement.

In general, people with a known cause for their hydrocephalus — trauma, for example — have a better chance of treatment success. So do those who have experienced signs and symptoms for only a short time. In some situations, your doctor may conduct a trial test before placing a permanent shunt, to see if you'll respond to fluid drainage. This can be done by draining fluid via spinal taps over several months and monitoring your improvement.

Huntington's disease

This progressive neurodegenerative disorder is characterized by uncontrolled movements, emotional disturbances and mental deterioration. Huntington's disease (Huntington's chorea) is an inherited disease. Signs and symptoms usually develop in middle age, and men are as likely as women to develop the condition. Younger adults with Huntington's disease often have more severe symptoms, and these symptoms may progress more quickly. In rare instances, children develop this condition.

An estimated one in 10,000 Americans has Huntington's disease, with about 30,000 known cases in the United States. About 150,000 Americans may be at risk of inheriting Huntington's disease.

Signs and symptoms
The earliest signs and symptoms of Huntington's disease are associated with emotional changes such as irritability, anger, paranoia or signs of depression. Decreased cognitive abilities include difficulties with making decisions, learning new information, responding to questions and remembering facts.

Early physical signs and symptoms of Huntington's disease may include mild balance problems, clumsiness and involuntary facial movements such as grimacing. As the disease progresses, other signs and symptoms develop, including sudden jerky, involuntary movements (chorea) throughout the body; a wide, prancing gait; halting or slurred speech; and dementia.

Huntington's disease usually develops slowly, and the severity of the problems is related to the degree of neuron loss. Death occurs about 10 to 30 years after the signs and symptoms first appear. Typically, the earlier symptoms appear, the faster the disease will progress. Death is often caused by a pneumonia-related infection or injuries related to a fall and its complications.

Screening and diagnosis
Huntington's disease results from a single abnormal gene on chromosome 4. Normally, this gene controls the production of a protein called huntingtin — note the difference in spelling between the protein and the disease. It's uncertain what the normal function of this gene is, but it's possible that the mutated gene produces a toxic form of huntingtin, leading to the destruction of nerve cells in the brain.

To determine whether symptoms are caused by Huntington's disease, your doctor performs a physical exam and obtains your medical history and a medical history of the family. He or she may ask about any recent emotional or intellectual changes that have occurred. A computerized tomography (CT) or magnetic resonance imaging (MRI) scan may show any changes to the brain's structure, reflecting the loss of neurons.

A blood test is available to determine whether a person carries the defective gene. Your doctor may suggest this test to confirm that the signs and symptoms are caused by Huntington's disease. Some people with a family history of the disease choose to take the test even before any symptoms develop, to determine whether they carry the defective gene.

Deciding whether to be tested early for the gene is a personal decision. If you're uncertain about whether to have the test, consider contacting a genetic counselor. Doctors who specialize in medical

genetics can help you weigh the pros and cons of testing, understand the implications of a positive or negative result, and walk
you through the testing process. If you choose to be tested, consider
paying for it with your own money so that the test results remain
within in your control.

Treatment

No treatment is available currently that can stop or reverse the
development of Huntington's disease, but several approaches can
be used to manage the signs and symptoms.

Antipsychotic drugs such as haloperidol can help control uncontrolled movements, violent outbursts and hallucinations.
Antipsychotics aren't prescribed in the presence of dystonia —
abrupt muscle contractions that may be caused by Huntington's —
as these medications may worsen the contractions, causing stiffness
and rigidity. Preliminary studies suggest that newer types of
antipsychotics, such as olanzapine and quetiapine, may be more
effective and cause fewer side effects.

Tranquilizers such as clonazepam can lessen anxiety. Various
antidepressants, including fluoxetine (Prozac, Sarafem), sertraline
(Zoloft) and nortriptyline (Aventyl, Pamelor), can help control
depression and the obsessive-compulsive rituals that some people
with Huntington's disease develop. Medications such as lithium
can help control extreme emotions and mood swings.

Psychotherapy, physical therapy and speech therapy also may
be helpful, particularly in the early stages of Huntington's disease.
These therapies may reduce the risk of the side effects associated
with the medications listed above and, at the same time, greatly
improve the person's quality of life.

People with Huntington's disease may burn as many as 5,000
calories a day. Therefore, it's important that they get adequate
nutrition and that they maintain a healthy body weight. They may
require assistance with meals. Allow plenty of time for eating.
Cutting food into small pieces or serving puréed food may make
it easier for the person to swallow and avoid choking. Extra vitamins and supplements may be a consideration, but check with
your doctor first.

Creutzfeldt-Jakob disease

Creutzfeldt-Jakob disease (CJD) is a degenerative brain disorder that affects about one person in a million worldwide. It's believed to occur when misshapen brain proteins (prions) attack brain cells, creating sponge-like holes in brain tissue. CJD typically occurs around the age of 60. Once a person becomes sick, the course of the disease is swift. He or she usually dies from complications of CJD within months of developing the first symptoms. Currently no treatment is able to stop or slow progression of the disease.

CJD captured the public eye in the 1990s when a form of the disease — named variant CJD (vCJD) — developed among a number of people in Great Britain who had eaten contaminated beef from cows that had bovine spongiform encephalopathy, the medical term for mad cow disease.

CJD and its variants belong to a broad group of diseases known as transmissible spongiform encephalopathies. The name derives from the fact that disease can be transmitted from animal to animal or animal to human, and from the appearance of spongy holes, visible under a microscope, in affected brain tissue.

Signs and symptoms

The main characteristic of Creutzfeldt-Jakob disease is the rapidly progressing symptoms of dementia. In the beginning, a person with CJD may experience:
- Problems with muscle coordination
- Personality changes
- Insomnia
- Blurred vision
- Unusual sensations, such as a sense that skin is sticky

The symptoms become dramatically worse, resulting in severe mental impairment. The person may develop involuntary muscle jerks, difficulty moving and speaking, and blindness.

Many people with CJD eventually fall into a coma. Heart failure, respiratory failure, pneumonia or other infections are generally the cause of death. The disease usually runs its course in about five to seven months after signs and symptoms first appear.

The variant of CJD associated with mad cow disease usually begins with psychiatric symptoms, such as depression, anxiety, apathy and delusions. Cognitive impairment occurs in the later stages. The variant affects people at a younger age than standard CJD does, and has a slightly longer duration — 12 to 14 months.

Causes

Prion proteins occur naturally in the brains of humans and animals. Normally they're harmless but, when misshapen, they can cause disease. They perform their intended function once they're folded into a specific three-dimensional shape. Most proteins fold spontaneously during or just after they're synthesized inside cells.

Protein folding isn't foolproof, however, and many proteins made by the body aren't usable. The rejects are sent to a kind of recycling center, where they're prepared for reuse. But as people age, the recycling process may stop working efficiently. As a result, misfolded proteins accumulate, causing serious problems.

Misshapen prions may enter brain cells and force normal proteins to misfold as well. The infected cells die. Eventually, large clusters of cells die, leaving the brain riddled with holes.

How do you get CJD?

Researchers have identified three basic ways that Creutzfeldt-Jakob disease may develop:

Spontaneously. Most people with CJD develop the disease for no apparent reason. This type of sporadic CJD accounts for more than 85 percent of all cases, although some may be due to unidentified contamination or genetic mutation during a person's lifetime.

By genetic mutation. In the United States, about 5 percent to 10 percent of people with CJD have a family history of the disease or test positive for a genetic mutation associated with CJD.

By contamination. The risk of being exposed to contamination with CJD-related prions is low. CJD can't be transmitted through air or casual contact such as touching. A small number of people have developed the disease after being exposed to infected human tissue as a result of medical procedures such as skin transplants or injections of contaminated growth hormone. (Since 1985, all human growth hormone in the United States is genetically re-engineered, eliminating the risk of CJD.)

Misshapen prions aren't affected by standard sterilization methods including heat, radiation, alcohol, benzene and formaldehyde. As a result, there's a very slight risk that instruments used in some types of brain surgery can harbor small bits of infected tissue.

Studies done in animals suggest that contaminated blood and related products may transmit the disease, but no case of a blood transfusion leading to CJD has been recorded in humans. So far, the CJD variant described above has been linked primarily to the consumption of beef infected with mad cow disease.

CJD and vCJD have long incubation periods, which means the disease won't show up until years after initial protein abnormalities occur. For vCJD, the incubation period is approximately 10 years.

Diagnosis

Doctors often can make an accurate diagnosis based on medical and personal histories, a neurological exam, and other diagnostic tests. The diagnostic process often requires eliminating other possible causes of the person's signs and symptoms.

MRI scans can show subtle, yet characteristic, abnormalities. Brain wave tests (electroencephalograms, or EEGs) also show a characteristic series of irregular brain waves referred to as "periodic complexes," although these are not seen in everyone with CJD.

The presence of a particular protein in cerebrospinal fluid may help confirm CJD in someone who is already showing signs and symptoms of the disease. Samples of spinal fluid can be obtained through a spinal tap (lumbar puncture).

Only a brain biopsy or an examination of brain tissue after death can confirm the presence of Creutzfeldt-Jakob disease.

Treatment

No effective treatment exists for either CJD or vCJD. A number of drugs have been tested — including steroids, antibiotics and antiviral agents — with disappointing results. For that reason, doctors focus on alleviating pain and other symptoms and on making people with these diseases as comfortable as possible.

Dementia associated with other disorders

Sometimes dementia can be the result of brain damage caused by a chronic disorder affecting other parts of the body. You may hear these cases referred to as secondary dementias, because the dementia develops as a complication of a disease that's characterized primarily by other symptoms.

Some of the conditions in which this may occur are Parkinson's disease, progressive supranuclear palsy, HIV/AIDS, multiple sclerosis and Wilson's disease.

Parkinson's disease dementia

Some people with Parkinson's disease may develop dementia in the later stages of their illness. Parkinson's disease is a disorder that affects mainly neurons producing dopamine, a neurotransmitter controlling muscle movement. People with Parkinson's often experience trembling, muscle rigidity, difficulty walking, and problems with balance and coordination. These symptoms generally develop after age 50, although the disease affects a small percentage of younger adults as well.

Symptoms of cognitive impairment may be present when a diagnosis of Parkinson's disease is made, but these are generally mild. Scientists have estimated that these symptoms develop into severe dementia in 30 percent to 40 percent of people with Parkinson's disease. However, the risk of a person with Parkinson's developing dementia increases with age. A recent study suggests that the overall prevalence of dementia in people with Parkinson's may be much greater — closer to 70 percent — especially as people with Parkinson's live longer and dementia is better understood.

Signs and symptoms. Parkinson's disease dementia may be characterized by the following signs and symptoms, some of which may fluctuate in intensity:

Impaired executive functions. These functions include the ability to plan, organize and problem-solve, as well as to understand complex concepts and follow internal cues for behavior.

Attention difficulties. A person with Parkinson's disease dementia may have difficulty paying attention or staying focused.

Memory problems. An ability to store new information may be retained, but accessing that information can be a challenge. Thus, a person with Parkinson's disease dementia may have difficulty remembering things unless given a visual or verbal cue. General forgetfulness is not as severe as it is with Alzheimer's disease.

Psychotic symptoms. Hallucinations similar to those experienced in dementia with Lewy bodies are a common symptom of Parkinson's disease dementia. They usually involve vivid, colorful images of people or animals, although sounds are not included. Delusions and paranoia are less common symptoms.

Causes. The cause of dementia in people with Parkinson's disease is a matter of considerable debate. Because Parkinson's disease dementia is so similar to dementia with Lewy bodies (see Chapter 8), some experts believe both disorders may be part of the same disease spectrum. Currently the only difference between a diagnosis of Parkinson's disease dementia and dementia with Lewy bodies is timing of the onset of symptoms. If motor deficits occur more

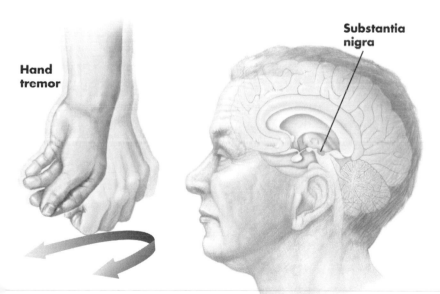

Substantia nigra

Hand tremor

Parkinson's disease

Movement problems associated with Parkinson's disease, such as tremor, are caused primarily by inadequate levels of the brain chemical dopamine, which transmits messages from the substantia nigra to other parts of the brain.

than a year before the cognitive difficulties begin, the disorder is considered to be Parkinson's disease dementia. If cognitive impairment occurs within a year of motor deficits, the diagnosis becomes dementia with Lewy bodies.

Lewy bodies — the name for abnormal deposits of the protein alpha-synuclein — are present in the brains of most people with Parkinson's disease. When there's no dementia involved, the Lewy bodies are restricted to an area of the brain called the substantia nigra. (For location of the substantia nigra, see page 163.) In people with Parkinson's disease dementia, Lewy bodies are found in other parts of the brain — areas associated with intellectual skills and emotions. A prominent theory is that the presence of Lewy bodies in these areas is what causes the dementia in Parkinson's disease. New information continues to emerge, however, suggesting that Lewy bodies may not be the only factor involved.

In addition, at autopsy, people with Parkinson's disease dementia frequently show amyloid plaques and neurofibrillary tangles. This implies that Alzheimer's disease may be a cause of the dementia and raises the possibility that Alzheimer's and Parkinson's are in some way connected.

It's also possible that the loss of dopamine-producing neurons, the main mechanism underlying Parkinson's disease, may itself cause or at least contribute to cognitive impairment and dementia, in spite of the Lewy bodies and Alzheimer's pathology.

Treatment. People with Parkinson's disease dementia experience a heavy loss of cholinergic neurons — neurons that produce acetylcholine — in addition to the loss of dopamine-producing neurons. In fact, the decrease in levels of acetylcholine, a characteristic of Alzheimer's disease, is far greater in people with Parkinson's disease dementia than in people with Alzheimer's. Preliminary studies indicate that cholinesterase inhibitors, medications that increase the level of acetylcholine in the brain, may be of some benefit for improving cognitive symptoms, although more research is needed to confirm these results.

Newer types of antipsychotic medications — quetiapine is commonly used — may help reduce hallucinations and other psychotic symptoms, with few side effects.

Progressive supranuclear palsy

A disorder that's often misdiagnosed as Parkinson's disease is progressive supranuclear palsy. It has many characteristics that are similar to those of Parkinson's disease such as an unsteady gait, stooped posture, muscle rigidity and difficulty with spoken language and articulation.

People with progressive supranuclear palsy have a tendency to fall backwards. They also have a greatly reduced rate of blinking, which often leads to dry eyes and increased susceptibility to eye infections. Eye movements in general become slowed. A characteristic symptom is an inability to focus the gaze downward.

About 15 percent of people with progressive supranuclear palsy develop some form of cognitive impairment. These problems may range from memory loss and personality changes to apathy, depression and anxiety. People with progressive supranuclear palsy often have difficulty with planning, organizing, decision making and abstract reasoning. Other signs and symptoms may include increased irritability, occasional angry outbursts and unexplained episodes of laughing or crying.

The destruction of neurons in the brain is far more widespread in progressive supranuclear palsy than it is in Parkinson's disease. The cause of the disease is undetermined, but like a number of other disorders — including Alzheimer's disease, frontotemporal dementia and corticobasal degeneration — it's characterized by the accumulation of tau protein deposits or neurofibrillary tangles. The relationship among various tau-related diseases, or tauopathies as they're sometimes called, is still not understood. But learning how to prevent tau accumulations in general may lead toward better treatments of these specific diseases.

At present, treatment of progressive supranuclear palsy is geared toward improving comfort and quality of life. Medications used to treat other movement disorders may be of help temporarily. Glasses with prisms can improve a person's ability to see downward, and artificial tears may soothe dry eyes. After the onset of symptoms, the course of the disease runs an average of seven years. Death is usually caused by a pneumonia-related infection or the complications of a fall or reduced mobility.

HIV/AIDS

Some people infected with the human immunodeficiency virus (HIV) may develop dementia eventually. This occurrence is often referred to as HIV-associated dementia or AIDS dementia complex. Before the widespread use of aggressive antiretroviral treatment, known as highly active antiretroviral therapy (HAART), approximately 20 percent to 30 percent of people with HIV went on to develop some level of HIV-associated dementia. More recently, given the success of HAART, the incidence of dementia in HIV-infected adults has decreased to about 10 percent.

HIV-associated dementia generally is characterized by memory loss, reduced concentration, impaired judgment, personality changes, mood swings, anxiety and, occasionally, hallucinations, paranoia and delusions.

Each person experiences signs and symptoms at a different rate and with different severity. Some may have very mild cognitive impairment, while others may become severely demented.

What causes the deterioration of brain cells in a person with HIV infection isn't understood, but the onset of dementia is correlated with the number of cells infected by the virus. One theory, sometimes called the Trojan horse hypothesis, is that the virus enters the central nervous system as a hidden passenger in immune cells that have access to the brain. Once there, the virus-infected cells go on to infect other cells in the brain, replicating the virus many times over.

During diagnosis, doctors try to distinguish HIV-associated dementia from other treatable causes of dementia. These causes might include infections of the brain such as meningitis, nutritional deficiencies, medication side effects, and psychiatric illnesses such as depression and anxiety.

At the same time that it greatly reduces the quantity of infected cells in the body, HAART also decreases the risk of HIV-associated dementia. But another, milder form of cognitive impairment has been identified that may develop into dementia later, particularly as new treatments extend the life span of a person infected with HIV. Thus, researchers continue to search for ways to protect the brain from the effects of this viral infection.

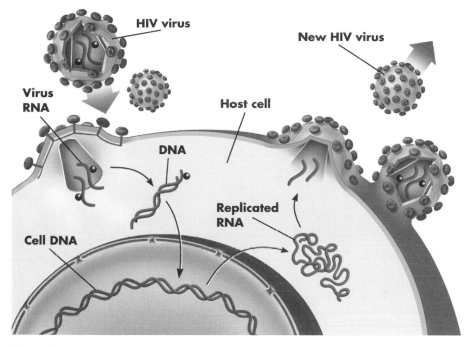

Human immunodeficiency virus (HIV) belongs to a family of viruses called retroviruses. These viruses carry their genetic information on single-stranded ribonucleic acid (RNA). Once inside a host cell, HIV is able to convert its RNA into double-stranded deoxyribonucleic acid (DNA). The viral DNA enters the nucleus and is inserted into the host cell's DNA. After this, HIV is able to replicate itself. When the cell bursts, the replicated viruses are released.

Multiple sclerosis

About half of all people with multiple sclerosis (MS) experience some degree of cognitive impairment. The impairment usually isn't as severe as it is in Alzheimer's disease and other forms of dementia, but it can affect a person's work life and social life and impair his or her daily living skills.

In multiple sclerosis, the body incorrectly directs antibodies and white blood cells to attack proteins in the myelin sheath, a protective coating that surrounds nerve fibers in your brain and spinal cord. This causes inflammation and injury to the sheath and ultimately to the nerves that it surrounds and protects. The result may be multiple areas of scarring (sclerosis). Eventually this damage slows or blocks the nerve signals that control muscle coordination, strength, sensation and vision.

In multiple sclerosis, the different types of cognitive impairment are believed to result from damage to nerves deep in the brain's white matter. Signs and symptoms may include:

- Difficulty remembering things without a reminder
- General forgetfulness
- Slowed reaction time
- Difficulty with planning, organizing, decision making and abstract reasoning
- Personality changes that include carelessness, irritability, lack of judgment and lack of responsiveness
- Difficulty with words
- Depression

These signs and symptoms generally occur in episodes (attacks) that last for weeks or months and are separated by periods in which the problems improve or disappear (remission). The types of

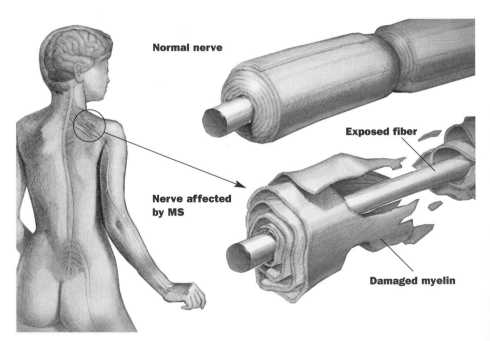

In multiple sclerosis, the protective coating on nerve fibers (myelin) becomes detached and eventually destroyed. Depending on where the nerve damage occurs, MS can affect vision, sensation, coordination, movement, and bladder and bowel control.

symptoms and their severity roughly correlate to the areas of the brain that are affected and to the degree of nerve damage. Cognitive symptoms are more likely to occur in people with a chronic, progressive form of multiple sclerosis.

Treatment of the underlying cause, multiple sclerosis, can help reduce the amount of new nerve damage and prevent or minimize associated cognitive decline. Studies suggest that some medications used to treat Alzheimer's may be beneficial in treating cognitive symptoms associated with MS, but more studies are needed to confirm the drug's efficacy and safety.

Wilson's disease

Wilson's disease is a hereditary disorder that causes too much of the mineral copper to accumulate in your liver, brain and other vital organs. Bile, a fluid that assists in digestion, normally carries excess copper away from your liver. In someone with Wilson's disease, the liver doesn't release the mineral into bile as it should. The resulting buildup of copper in the liver injures the tissue. Eventually, some of the excess copper travels throughout the body, where it may damage your brain, eyes, kidneys and red blood cells. If left untreated, Wilson's disease is fatal.

In some people, Wilson's disease can cause abrupt personality changes and inappropriate social behavior. Tremors, muscle spasms and speech problems also may occur. Later complications of the disease include mood swings, depression, agitation, loss of memory and periods of confusion.

With early diagnosis and treatment, the progression of the disease can be stopped, and existing symptoms may be improved. Treatment involves taking medications that either remove the deposited copper from tissues or render it harmless. The two medications approved for this purpose are penicillamine (Cuprimine, Depen) and trientine (Syprine). Taking zinc acetate (Galzin) helps block copper absorption from the stomach and intestine and may be an alternative treatment for pregnant women and people without symptoms or organ damage. Although treatment is lifelong, the long-term outlook and life expectancy are generally good for people with Wilson's disease.

Many causes

Like a finely tuned machine, your brain depends on a harmonious balance among all of its parts for efficient operation. Even a slight disruption in this balance may have serious consequences. As described in previous chapters, your brain and nervous system are vulnerable to a wide variety of injuries. Degeneration of nerve cells causes illnesses such as Alzheimer's disease. Interruption of the blood supply to the brain causes strokes.

The conditions described in this chapter provide a broader picture of the many cognitive disorders that can affect or destroy mental processing and learning. The causes range from genetic mutation and abnormal protein to chemical imbalance and a buildup of cerebrospinal fluid that cushions the brain.

Neurologists and other medical specialists must try to determine a cause and prescribe appropriate treatment. Diagnosis may be difficult because signs and symptoms are so numerous and diverse. And many of the signs and symptoms can be associated with cognitive loss in general and are not exclusive to a specific condition. A careful assessment of the character and pattern of signs and symptoms over time, in addition to laboratory tests, are sometimes necessary to reach an accurate diagnosis.

Part 4

Expanding knowledge of dementia

Research in recent years is starting to
push open doors that block understanding of dementia. Some of the biggest
advances have focused on the earliest stages,
and even the pre-stages, of the disorder, when
it's hoped that dementia is most treatable.

Chapter 11

Mild cognitive impairment

Medical experts emphasize that a dementing disorder such as Alzheimer's disease doesn't start all of a sudden, with little warning. Its onset is gradual, with mild symptoms developing into more severe ones in the disease process. This transition from mild to severe is thought to exist on a continuum. The dictionary defines *continuum* as "a continuous whole," in this case, a variety of signs and symptoms that overlap and interconnect, progressively eroding away a person's cognitive functions.

Recent research has focused on the mild end of this continuum and the concept of a dementia prodrome — warning signs indicating the transition between normal cognition and the early stages of dementia. The term commonly used for this transition stage is mild cognitive impairment (MCI).

In general, mild cognitive impairment is characterized by subtle difficulties with certain aspects of cognition even while other aspects of cognition remain relatively normal. A person with mild cognitive impairment may experience new, deteriorating patterns of forgetfulness, yet still be able to handle his or her finances, perform household tasks capably and drive a car with few problems. This person may have developed memory loss that is more severe than what occurs in the "normal" aging described in Chapter 2, but not so severe as to be classified as dementia.

Researchers have taken a keen interest in this concept of a pre-dementia stage because, if the ability to diagnose a disease such as Alzheimer's in its earliest phase is developed, it opens up the possibility of new therapies that can arrest the disease process before severe, irreversible damage occurs to the brain.

The concept of this distinct transition stage is still evolving. Doctors have yet to agree on the precise criteria that determine whether a person has mild cognitive impairment — the signs and symptoms may appear in different ways and at different times. In addition, the mechanisms underlying the impairment are still undetermined and may vary.

Of greatest significance perhaps to scientists is that not everyone diagnosed with mild cognitive impairment goes on to develop dementia. For sure, the presence of mild cognitive impairment signals an increased risk of dementia, but some individuals remain stable while others revert to a normal cognitive status. In other words, the dementia continuum doesn't appear to be in one direction at early stages — it doesn't point just from mild to severe.

Nonetheless, as research data begin to consolidate and reveal characteristic patterns, an understanding of this transition stage will no doubt contribute clues to the way in which dementia develops, particularly in the case of Alzheimer's disease. These findings may greatly extend the options for diagnosis and treatment of many other cognitive disabilities.

Subcategories of MCI

Mild cognitive impairment is a term that encompasses a wide range of variation in what people experience. At present, two broad categories of mild cognitive impairment have been identified, based on the predominant signs and symptoms: amnestic MCI and non-amnestic MCI.

Amnestic MCI
Stemming from the word *amnesia*, amnestic MCI is characterized primarily by memory impairment. Abnormalities in other cognitive

areas, such as attention, language use and the processing speed of mental activity, may exist, but these symptoms usually are extremely mild and may not even be noticeable to the person or to observers. The person is likely to be living independently and functioning well within his or her community. Worries about newly developed (or worsening) forgetfulness are the most likely reasons for someone at this stage to want to see a doctor.

When tested for memory skills, the person doesn't perform as well as his or her peers of similar age and education, but the impairment doesn't meet the standard criteria for Alzheimer's disease. If only memory impairment is present, then the condition is classified as amnestic MCI-single domain. If other areas of cognitive impairment are detected in addition to memory impairment — for example, difficulties with language, concentration or visuospatial skills — then the classification is amnestic MCI-multiple domain. For example, a person may experience forgetfulness in addition to taking longer to perform simple household tasks and having difficulty with concentration.

Amnestic MCI is the most common form of mild cognitive impairment and also is the most studied and discussed in medical literature. Generally, it's believed that amnestic MCI is caused by a neurodegenerative disorder such as Alzheimer's.

Nonamnestic MCI

This subcategory of MCI applies to a person who experiences difficulty in a cognitive area other than memory, such as executive skills — for example, reasoning and judgment — or language and communication skills.

Researchers hypothesize that the development of a mild yet persistent problem with executive skills may represent the early stages of a non-Alzheimer's type of dementia such as frontotemporal dementia. They also believe that development of mild language difficulties may be linked to primary progressive aphasia, a type of dementia that primarily affects language skills.

As with amnestic MCI, only one cognitive skill may be affected (nonamnestic MCI-single domain) or multiple skills are affected (nonamnestic MCI-multiple domain).

Mild cognitive impairment

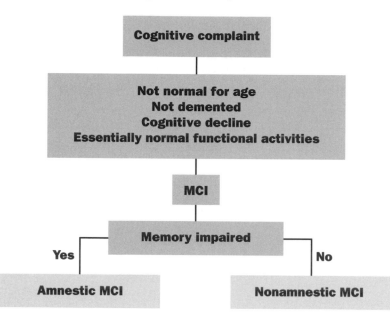

This flowchart shows the decision process your doctor would follow to make a diagnosis of mild cognitive impairment.

Causes

For either subcategory of MCI, there may be more than one underlying cause. The various causes generally are grouped into one of the following categories:

Neurodegenerative. A disorder that gradually destroys brain cells (for example, Alzheimer's disease, dementia with Lewy bodies or frontotemporal dementia)

Vascular. A disorder that affects the blood vessels of the brain and the supply of oxygen and nutrients vital to brain cells, causing cell damage and death (vascular cognitive impairment)

Psychiatric. Certain psychiatric conditions that affect memory, concentration and mood (for example, depression)

Trauma. Physical injury to the brain that also may lead to cognitive difficulties — the potential cause, such as a severe blow to the head, is usually obvious

Potential outcomes of MCI

Syndrome	Causes		
	Neurodegenerative	**Vascular**	**Psychiatric**
Amnestic MCI			
Single domain	Alzheimer's		Depression
Multiple domain	Alzheimer's	Vascular cognitive impairment	Depression
Nonamnestic MCI			
Single domain	Frontotemporal dementia		Attention deficit disorder
Multiple domain	Dementia with Lewy bodies	Vascular cognitive impairment	

Diagnosis

Criteria have been proposed for the diagnosis of mild cognitive impairment, based on the results of various research studies. The criteria include:

- A new cognitive complaint, usually memory loss, that's growing more frequent or more severe, preferably corroborated by a family member or friend
- Generally normal function of other cognitive activity
- Generally normal participation in the activities of daily living, including household duties, work and social functions
- Cognitive impairment is determined when compared objectively with others of a similar age (as measured by neuropsychological testing)
- No dementia is noted

In practice, the diagnosis of MCI can be a challenge. A memory complaint is often subjective, based on the degree to which a person feels it impacts his or her daily life — and that assessment varies considerably from one individual to the next. Furthermore, the person must be aware of the memory difficulties in order to make the complaint — which sometimes doesn't happen. In this sense, corroboration of the events from someone who knows the person well can be very helpful.

Usually, the complaint will be a new pattern of forgetfulness, such as a difficulty remembering appointments or important dates and names that once were easy to remember. In other words, the occasional forgetting of an appointment is fairly normal, but regular memory slip-ups in your routine may be a sign of a more serious underlying problem.

Once a cognitive problem is brought to a doctor's attention, the doctor will conduct an extensive interview to gather information about the incidents and about the person's history. The doctor will also conduct a mental status evaluation to assess the evidence of any cognitive decline. If there appears to be a greater degree of change than is warranted for someone of that age — but still not reaching the level of dementia — the doctor may suspect a development of mild cognitive impairment.

Neuropsychological testing can help determine whether the person's memory or other cognitive functions is impaired when compared with others in his or her age group. But currently there's no established dividing line or an accepted set of markers that determine who has MCI and who doesn't. As a result, diagnosis is partly dependent on the doctor's judgment, within the context of an individual case. In general, an experienced physician will rely on a combination of personal interviews, medical history and clinical test results to identify any changes in cognition, rather than simply relying on test scores from the evaluation, to make a diagnosis.

If memory is impaired but other cognitive skills — attention span, language use, concentration, reasoning and judgment — remain relatively unaffected, then a diagnosis of amnestic MCI-single domain may be made. If multiple cognitive skills are affected, then the diagnosis may be one of amnestic MCI-multiple domain. By the same token, an impairment of a cognitive skill other than memory may lead to a diagnosis of nonamnestic MCI, further classified as single domain or multiple domain, depending on the number of cognitive skills affected.

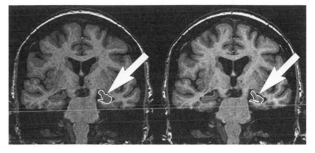

These MRIs show the same individual as normal (left) and diagnosed later with MCI (right). The image on the right shows the hippocampus (circled white) has shrunken slightly.

Brain imaging tests

Advances in brain imaging have allowed scientists to gather data about the hippocampus — a structure of the brain important in memory. Studies using magnetic resonance imaging (MRI) indicate that the volume of the hippocampus is frequently smaller in people who progress from MCI to dementia than in those with MCI who don't go on to develop dementia. As such, refined measurements of the hippocampus may, at some point, be used as a predictive tool for risk in people who have been diagnosed with MCI.

Scientists are studying other forms of brain imaging that may prove helpful in diagnosing mild cognitive impairment and in distinguishing those individuals at higher risk of dementia. Studies of functional neuroimaging — imaging that evaluates the activity of the brain rather than its physical structure — indicate that certain changes in brain activity may accompany the onset of mild cognitive impairment. These changes may end up potentially serving as markers for increased risk of Alzheimer's.

For example, a type of stain called Pittsburgh Compound B (PIB) has been developed that readily sticks to clumps of amyloid beta (plaques) in the living brain. The stain pattern can be seen with the use of a brain imaging technique called positron emission tomography (PET). This new compound may allow physicians to monitor the amount of amyloid beta in the brain and note the development of plaques, potentially helping to confirm a diagnosis of MCI. For more on this technique, see Chapter 13.

When preventive treatments for dementia are discovered and become readily available, it will be important to identify people with a higher risk of developing dementia, as they will be the ones most likely to benefit from treatment.

Outcome

Long-term studies indicate that people with mild cognitive impairment, particularly amnestic MCI, are at an increased risk of Alzheimer's disease — they tend to develop the dementia at a much higher rate than the general population that does not have MCI. Exactly how many people with MCI go on to develop Alzheimer's, and the rate at which this progression occurs, is the subject of much ongoing research. The numbers vary from study to study, at least in part due to varying criteria for identifying MCI.

The Mayo Alzheimer's Disease Research Center followed a group of individuals with amnestic MCI from the time of their registry as patients for a period of three to six years. Within this group, the rate of progression to dementia was within the range of 10 percent to 15 percent a year. Other studies have shown similar results. Among older adults with no MCI, progression to dementia is about 1 percent to 2 percent a year.

The Mayo data suggest that about 80 percent of people who meet the criteria for amnestic MCI would develop Alzheimer's within six years. It also indicates that people carrying the apolipoprotein ε4 (APOE ε4) variation in their genes were likely to progress more rapidly than people who didn't have the variation. (See Chapter 5 for more information on this gene.)

An ongoing long-term study of aging and Alzheimer's disease in a group of older Catholic clergy yielded information about the course of mild cognitive impairment over a follow-up period of four and one-half years. This clergy had agreed to annual evaluations as well as postmortem brain donation. From among nearly 800 participants, just over 200 were diagnosed as having mild cognitive impairment. The study found that those with mild cognitive impairment were three times more likely to develop Alzheimer's than those with no mild cognitive impairment.

In a community-based study of over 1,200 older adults who had no dementia on enrollment, approximately 3 percent to 4 percent were found to have developed amnestic MCI over the course of the study. The participants were evaluated every two years for a period of 10 years. Of those with amnestic MCI:

- Between 10 percent and 17 percent progressed to Alzheimer's disease every two years. In this study, people with MCI had four times the risk of developing Alzheimer's as people with no cognitive impairment.
- Up to 5 percent progressed to non-Alzheimer forms of dementia.
- Between 10 percent and 20 percent of participants remained stable with MCI — with cognitive functions getting neither better or worse.
- Between one-third and one-half of participants either improved or reverted to normal, worsened but didn't become demented, or had mixed results.

In addition, the development of new cases of mild cognitive impairment among participants over the course of this study was 2 percent to 3 percent.

Other studies report variations on these figures, but in general most studies confirm the idea of mild cognitive impairment as a distinct stage that puts you at high risk of dementia.

Inside the MCI brain

Scientists are beginning to investigate the pathological changes that may be occurring in the brain of a person with MCI. How does the brain function at the stage when cognitive impairment is just starting? A detailed answer to this question is a firm step toward understanding the early stages of dementia and providing new opportunities for diagnosis and treatment.

What researchers have discovered so far is that the brain of a person with MCI doesn't show the heavy load of plaques and tangles that are known to be present in the Alzheimer's brain. However, certain disease-related changes have begun to occur, particularly in sections of the temporal lobes — areas of the brain vital to memory and learning.

Although several findings have cast an interesting light on the question, the manner in which these bits of knowledge fit within the big picture is not yet clear. These findings include:

- Autopsies performed on people diagnosed with MCI reveal a strong association between levels of cognitive impairment and distributions of neurofibrillary tangles in the brain.
- On the other hand, when the densities of amyloid plaques are analyzed at autopsies, the MCI brain appears more similar to a normal brain than to an Alzheimer's brain — meaning many fewer plaques are present.
- In addition, there's evidence of non-Alzheimer's disorders in the MCI brain, including a strong presence of vascular disease.

Based on this current research, it appears that, pathologically, Alzheimer's disease or another form of dementia has not fully developed in the brain of a person with MCI. This would indicate the possibility of being able to intervene early in the disease process and preventing the disorder from advancing.

Treatment

Most research suggests that by the time a person is diagnosed with Alzheimer's disease, it's too late to stop the disorder or reverse the damage that's been done. Focusing on mild cognitive impairment as a likely precursor to Alzheimer's may lead to strategies that help prevent or delay progression of the disease. Several studies are under way to evaluate the effects of different compounds introduced to the brain during the transition from mild cognitive impairment to Alzheimer's.

As a starting point, most researchers are examining drugs or other compounds that have already shown some effect on Alzheimer's disease. One of the primary research targets is cholinesterase inhibitors. These drugs have been approved by the Food and Drug Administration (FDA) for Alzheimer's and have been shown to help stabilize cognitive function in the disease's early stages by increasing brain levels of acetlycholine. Acetlycholine is a chemical that typically decreases in the disease process. These drugs include donepezil (Aricept), rivastigmine (Exelon) and galantamine (Razadyne, formerly known as Reminyl). (For more on these medications and how they work, see Chapter 6).

Other potential therapies being considered for MCI are similar to others being explored for Alzheimer's (for more information, see Chapter 13), including:

Antioxidants. Substances such as vitamin E, gingko biloba and selegeline may protect brain cells from the oxidative stress that appears to play a role in Alzheimer's

Anti-inflammatory agents. Medications such as nonsteroidal anti-inflammatory drugs (NSAIDs) may help to reduce inflammation in the brain

Drugs that alter brain chemical levels. Dopamine agonists and glutamate receptor antagonists may be used in an attempt to normalize the effects of the disease process

The vitamin E and donepezil

In 2005, results were published from a large study comparing the effects of vitamin E, donepezil and a placebo (inactive pill) on people with amnestic MCI over a period of three years. The study enrolled well over 700 participants. Of these, just over 200 developed Alzheimer's during the trial at a rate of 16 percent per year.

In the study, vitamin E appeared to have no benefit in slowing the progression to Alzheimer's. On the other hand, people who received donepezil progressed at a slower rate than those in the vitamin E and the placebo groups for the first 12 months of the trial. By the end of trial, however, this effect had disappeared and there was no significant difference in the total number of people in each group who had developed Alzheimer's.

Researchers conducting the trial still aren't certain why donepezil worked only for a short term. They speculate that the drug's effects may have worn off after a period of time or that the burden of the disease gradually overtook the modest effects of the drug. Nonetheless, the fact that donepezil temporarily delayed the progression to Alzheimer's disease is incentive to pursue further studies in treating mild cognitive impairment.

The study revealed a number of complex results that scientists are sorting through. For example, the study confirmed previous findings that the APOE ε4 genetic variant was an important risk factor for Alzheimer's — three-quarters of the people who progressed from MCI to Alzheimer's were APOE ε4 carriers. The effects of donepezil, however, appeared to last the longest among this group of APOE ε4 carriers, reducing their risk of Alzheimer's by about a third for most of the study.

Not enough is known about this aspect of Alzheimer's to recommend that people be tested for this genetic variation, but it does provide material for future study. It may be that treatments for cognitive impairment will be designed according to a person's genetic profile, not unlike other diseases where a particular gene represents increased risk, such as the BRCA gene in breast cancer.

Making progress

More than anything, the vitamin E and donepezil study shows that treatment of mild cognitive impairment is a viable starting point for fighting Alzheimer's disease and, possibly, other forms of dementia. Most scientists are certain that preventive treatment for Alzheimer's will be developed in the next few decades. It stands to reason that identifying those at high risk of the disease, such as people with mild cognitive impairment, will be essential to deriving the maximum benefit from preventive treatment.

The challenge facing scientists who study MCI is twofold: one direction lies in further refining the parameters for diagnosing the condition and identifying those who will go on to develop dementia. The other lies in identifying and customizing treatments that will prevent mild cognitive impairment from progressing into dementia.

Chapter 12

Staying mentally sharp

It always seems to happen at the worst possible time. Forgetfulness can disrupt your daily routine and ruin an otherwise perfect moment. You spend 20 minutes in a frantic search for your glasses, only to find them resting on the top of your head. Or you get all the way to the grocery store or movie theater before you realize you left your pocketbook on the kitchen counter. And how many times have you momentarily laid something aside for safe keeping, only to forget where that safe place is?

Memory lapses such as these happen to just about everyone in certain situations and at certain times. For example, if you're a busy person with a full schedule, you may find yourself bombarded with a lot of details. These are ideal conditions for occasional memory lapses. The word *occasional* is key. Memory problems such as these usually aren't persistent — they may even disappear when you have fewer commitments.

Memory lapses are a common complaint of people age 50 and older, and often blamed on aging. Some older adults worry that this may signal the beginnings of dementia. But, as described in previous chapters of this book, dementia involves much more than occasional forgetfulness. The symptoms of dementia affect many aspects of your daily life — not just memory — and these symptoms progressively worsen.

Effects of aging on brain function

Will your mental abilities change as you age? Research indicates the answer is yes, they probably will. Based on some of the physiological changes described in Chapter 2, you may expect the following to typically occur in many older adults:

- It takes a little longer to learn new things. You either learn less in the same amount of time or need more time to learn the same amount, compared with when you were younger.
- It's harder to recall some names, faces, dates and other pieces of factual information.
- It's more difficult to handle multiple tasks at the same time. You may need to focus on only one task and accomplish it well before turning your attention to the next task.

Still, it's important to remember two key points. First, many factors besides age affect mental function. Depression and chronic stress are two of the most common factors. Both can cause difficulty with recent memory, decrease attention and concentration, and impair your ability to make decisions. The good news is that both conditions are treatable.

Second, no two people age in the same way. Your mental strengths and weaknesses as a young adult are likely to continue as you get older. For example, if you've always been good at remembering people's names, you're likely to continue to do well in that capacity. If you've always had trouble remembering names, you're not likely to get much better at it with age. In fact, this type of problem may even get worse.

Happily, most experts believe that something can be done to improve memory and reduce the occurrence of memory lapses. Older adults can learn just as well as younger adults, and it's possible to increase the number of brain cell connections, regardless of age. Certain lifestyle measures, such as being physically active, limiting alcohol use and managing stress, also have been shown to benefit mental function.

Perhaps the best way to keep your mind sharp is simply by exercising it. Just as regular physical activity such as walking improves your heart and lung capacity and gets you in shape, so mental activity can improve your brain function. These can be simple activities that you enjoy, such as reading, doing puzzles and games, and picking up a new hobby. Memory lapses may not disappear completely, but you're likely to have fewer of them.

Strategies for staying mentally sharp

Memory depends heavily on the physical and emotional makeup and social experience of each individual, but most people generally develop habits to help offset age-related changes. Even if research hasn't outlined all the ins and outs of human intellect, keeping your brain active and engaged in the world makes for a more interesting life — and who can resist that possibility?

Here are five practical strategies that may help you keep your brain in shape:

1. Use reminders to keep organized

In today's world, information bombards you from many directions. You need to get past the information overload. If you start developing habits that are helpful reminders at a younger age, you'll cope better as you get older — but it's never too late to start.

Keep track of necessary information. Most of the information you need to remember on your daily to-do list will probably fall into one of three categories:

- Scheduled appointments
- Tasks that need to get done, though not at a scheduled time
- Addresses, phone numbers and other contact information for the key people in your life

To get organized, develop methods to track each type of information. For example, list your scheduled appointments in a personal calendar. Create a list for unscheduled tasks. Maintain a file with the names, addresses and phone numbers of people you need to contact regularly. A wide variety of tools are available to help you organize, maintain and remember this information — ranging from simple paper records to sophisticated computer software. Even a simple list hung on the wall above the phone will help.

Set up a filing system. Buried in the stack of throw-away mail that you receive each week are bills, bank statements, meeting notices, and special announcements. Use the following tips to dig out the items worth retaining:

- *Tame the paper tiger.* Instead of letting paper accumulate in miscellaneous piles, sort mail and other documents as soon as you get them. As you sort, ask yourself: "Will I ever need this document again?" If the answer is yes, keep it. If the answer is no, throw it away.
- *File instead of pile.* Some documents contain information that you'll consult only occasionally. Examples are tax records; statements for your checking, savings and investment accounts; insurance policies and other key contracts; and owner's manuals for appliances, cars and other possessions. Create special files for these items. At least once a year, review these files and purge anything that's irrelevant.
- *Create a to-read file.* Gather magazines, newsletters and brochures that can be read at any time. Keep these items together and save them for bedtime reading or weekend relaxation or even your next plane trip.

2. Develop routines, rituals and cues

Like them or not, routines are invaluable for organizing your day. Store frequently used items in the same place, whether at work or at home. Try to carry your car keys or house keys in the same location whenever they're on you — always in the same pocket or handbag — and always return them to a designated spot when you're finished with them. Keep the kitchen utensils that you use for certain tasks together in convenient locations, for example, bowls with measuring cups or knives with cutting boards. Use a toolbox to store tools that you may need every once in a while, such as a hammer, pliers and wrench. Always put the tools back when you're done using them so you know where they are for the next time you need them.

Rituals are series of actions that you train yourself to do in a specific order (or at the same time). Rituals can ease the completion of many common tasks. For example, you might start a list of grocery items that you intend to buy at the beginning of each week and keep that list at a handy place in the kitchen. You schedule a shopping trip on a particular day and take that list out to your car first thing in the morning on that day. You shop at the same store each time so that you're familiar with the location of each item on the list. For another example, before leaving your house for an overnight trip, you check the house in a specific sequence: You make sure all appliances and lights are switched off, adjust the thermostat, lock the windows, then lock the garage door, side door and front door on your way out.

A cue is anything that signals you to do something, be it an object or a sound or even a smell. Many people like to place objects in uncommon locations in order to help them remember. For example, place letters to mail in your pathway to the front door so that you don't forget them as you leave the house. Many people stick reminder notes on the bathroom mirror or the refrigerator at night to make sure they'll do something the next morning. Some people depend on auditory cues, for example, setting their watch alarms a few minutes before appointments.

3. Use memory techniques

Studies on memory suggest a number of memory techniques may be useful aids. Experiment with the following techniques to see if one of them will work for you. Most prompt you to encode more efficiently — that is, to mentally focus on information when you first encounter it and to manipulate it in such a way that it helps you remember. Consider the use of a memory technique like the playing of a game — have fun with it.

Make associations. One way to remember something new is to associate it with something else that you already know. You did this as a child when you learned to recognize Italy on a world map by remembering that the country is shaped like a boot, or that the state of Michigan resembles a mitten.

Association can also work for learning definitions. For example, to remember that the port side of a boat is the left side (and not the right), remind yourself that the words *port* and *left* both have four letters — associating them — whereas as *right* has five letters.

You can apply association in more sophisticated ways. Say that you're trying to remember the name of a person you worked with 10 years ago and haven't seen since. If that name doesn't pop immediately into your mind, try to think of something associated with that person that you do remember. Visualize the building you both worked in, the location of your offices or the name of your supervisor. Prompting your memory with related details might yield the information you want.

In similar fashion, when receiving information that you'd like to remember, simply ask yourself certain questions that may prompt later associations. For example:

- How is the person I just met this morning similar to someone I already know well?
- How does this alternate route to downtown relate to the route I normally travel?
- How will this information help me accomplish the goal I've set out to accomplish?

Select your memories. Sometimes it's necessary to be selective about what you're trying to remember. Remind yourself of what's truly important and what's of less priority. When meeting many new people at the same time, for example, try to focus on retaining just a handful of key names — better to remember a few than to be confused about everyone. When reading a news article, give it a skim to consider what facts or ideas may be the most important to remember, then return for the full details.

To reinforce memories, continue to ask questions — this time to separate information you're sure you'll want to recall from information that you feel may be OK to forget:

- *What level of the ramp am I parked on?* If on the third level, you may say to yourself "triple crown" as a reminder. What car is parked beside mine? Don't worry — by the time you return, other vehicles will be in the adjoining spaces.
- *What landmarks do I need to remember on this route?* Count the number of intersections with stoplights or stop signs. Note any large or distinctive billboards. What's that music on the car radio? Enjoy the music but don't fiddle with tuning to new stations as you travel the route.

Repeat, rehash and revisit. Exercise your memory by retrieving key information often. Review the essential facts — names, dates, numbers — several times when you first try to learn them.

When you want to remember key concepts or ideas, talk about them and formulate your own opinions. To be able to recall the main ideas of a book you've just finished, for example, it helps to summarize them in a conversation with family or friends. The same technique applies for the plots of movies or for song lyrics.

You may want to review relevant information in advance of a special event — such as paging through your high school yearbook before attending a class reunion to remember names and faces.

Other memory techniques. Here are more strategies that may help you remember new information:

- *Break it down.* Divide new information into meaningful chunks. You do this already when you break down a ten-digit phone number, such as 8005551212, into the area code, three-digit exchange number and four-digit personal number: 800-555-1212. Apply the same technique to items such as a license plate number, social security number or computer password.

- *Pay attention.* Forgetfulness may just be a sign of mental overload. Slow down and pay full attention to the task at hand, whatever it may be. Reduce distractions, for example, by turning off the radio or TV while you're reading instructions. Control your work environment to reduce interruptions, such as shutting the office door when you need to concentrate on a report. Whenever possible, do one thing at a time.

- *Picture it.* Create a vivid mental image of the information you want to remember. To recall where information is stored on your personal computer, visualize a huge, virtual filing cabinet that contains folders and subfolders for your documents, carefully organized and color-coded by subject.

- *Write it down.* The act of writing involves mental actions that often stay with you. Writing a to-do list, for example, might help you remember your priorities for the day, even if you misplace the list. Recording a sequence of events and your feelings about them in a journal may help you remember the experience, even if you never reread the passage.

4. Don't be afraid of challenges

Although you may not be able to do some things as well as you did them before, age shouldn't stop you from pursuing new frontiers. Studies show that older adults learn new skills as well as younger adults do. While younger adults may be able to mentally process faster, older adults can apply more wisdom and experience.

Don't be afraid to test your limits. Excitement is an important part of learning. Former president George H. W. Bush celebrated his 75th birthday by skydiving. The first time he made a parachute jump was when his plane was shot down over the Pacific Ocean during World War II. After that experience, he promised himself he would one day jump out of a plane for fun.

Get creative. If you're not one for skydiving, creative work may be suitable. Artist Georgia O'Keefe, after discontinuing her work for years, returned to painting and sculpting at the age of 86 and went on to receive the Medal of the Arts. At 74, actor Clint Eastwood won an Oscar for directing "Million Dollar Baby," which also starred 68-year-old Morgan Freeman. Freeman beat out younger actors to win his own Oscar for best supporting actor. Even in his nineties, architect Philip Johnson continued to exert influence on the design and aesthetics of buildings. Quite simply, it's never too late to turn out some of your best work.

On the other hand, it doesn't take celebrity status to expand your horizons. Here are a few ways to get you started:

- Take adult or continuing education classes — learn yoga or Pilates or try your hand at painting or creative writing.
- Volunteer your skills or knowledge to the local school system or to a civic or charitable organization.
- Stay up-to-date on new technology, such as computers, cameras and telecommunications — you can do so cheaply by reading trade journals and visiting specialty stores.
- Stay in touch with family and friends and look to expand your circle of acquaintances.
- Join a book club or other discussion group.
- Attend local concerts, lectures and plays to explore the cultural life of your community.
- Research family history and publish your account.

The experience of age provides a rich backdrop for developing skills, embracing change and integrating knowledge into your life.

5. Take care of yourself

Caring for your body helps care for your mind. Being physically active, getting enough sleep, limiting alcohol and managing stress all contribute to keeping your brain at its optimum function.

Stay physically active. Even if it's just a short walk, physical activity improves blood flow and increases the supply of oxygen to the brain. Being active also reduces your risk of heart disease and stroke, which may reduce your risk of mental illness. It's possible that physical activity helps the brain by decreasing the harmful effects of certain hormones that affect your response to stress. Some research even suggests that physical activity may promote the regeneration of brain cells or the development of new ones.

One study, based on data from nearly 19,000 women between the ages of 70 and 81, showed that regular physical activity was associated with higher levels of mental functioning, an effect similar to being three years younger. The activity didn't have to be strenuous to have an effect: walking at least an hour and a half each week at a leisurely pace provided discernable mental benefits.

The same appears to be true for men. One study showed that older men who walked regularly were less likely to develop dementia. Another study found that participants who maintained or increased their physical activity over a period of 10 years had less mental decline.

Get a good night's rest. Sleep is one of life's basic necessities, right there at the top of the list with air, food and drink. A good night's sleep leaves you feeling refreshed, alert and ready to tackle the day ahead of you. On the other hand, sleep deprivation can lead to forgetfulness and problems with attention and concentration. You may feel less alert and vigorous, and more confused, irritable and fatigued.

Getting plenty of sleep sounds great, you may think, but as you get older, sleep just doesn't seem to come as easily as it did when you were younger. Unfortunately, for many, sleep tends to decrease and become less restful with age.

Limit alcohol. Excessive alcohol consumption can have immediate effects on your brain, causing poor concentration and judgment, and impaired motor skills. Heavy drinking has other long-term consequences. People who regularly drink to excess can experience permanent brain damage due to poor nutrition. They're also at higher risk of developing memory problems and dementia.

While it's true that moderate alcohol consumption can provide some health benefits, such as reducing your risk of heart disease, drinking too much quickly negates such benefits.

Manage stress. Studies show that chronic stress — the persistent feeling of being overwhelmed by life's challenges — can cause shrinkage of the hippocampus, an area of the brain important to the creation and storage of memories.

Research also suggests that how you respond to stress influences its impact on you. Stress itself isn't necessarily good or bad — the positive or negative effects depend on you and the amount of stress you're able to tolerate.

Acute stress — stress with an end in sight — can be mentally stimulating. These challenges include taking a test or giving a speech. A tolerable amount of stress can make these tasks exciting, whereas a lack of stress could seem downright boring.

Chronic stress — stress with no end in sight — has effects that can be harmful. It not only impairs cognitive processes but also over the long run can harm your immune system and lead to fatigue, depression, anxiety, anger and irritability.

One way to prevent chronic stress is to pursue positive and meaningful activities rather than those that saddle you with an unnecessary emotional load. Another way to cope with stress is to exercise, which can release tension in muscles, improve sleep and boost levels of endorphins — your body's natural painkillers.

Nature or Nurture?

It's a classic example of the chicken-and-egg syndrome. Scientists aren't sure whether brain power is responsible for intellectual achievements or whether intellectual achievements produce more brain power. Some experts maintain that an intellectually stimulating environment improves mental ability, even into old age. Much

Medications and your memory

If you've become concerned about memory lapses, ask your doctor about any side effects from the medications you may be taking. Some medications, including the examples below, can interfere with your ability to remember. When you talk to your doctor, mention everything you're taking, including vitamins, minerals, over-the-counter drugs and herbal supplements.

A couple of points to remember: Just because you're using one of the medications listed below doesn't mean that you're going to develop memory problems. In addition, some people may experience forgetfulness related to medications that aren't on this list.

Medications with possible memory side effects

Category	Generic name (brand name)
Anti-anxiety medications	• Alprazolam (Xanax) • Clonazepam (Klonopin) • Diazepam (Valium) • Lorazepam (Ativan)
Antidepressant medications	• Nortriptyline (Aventyl, Pamelor) • Amitriptyline • Imipramine (Tofranil)
Blood pressure medications	• Mexiletine (Mexitil) • Propranolol (Inderal)
Pain medications	• Fentanyl (Duragesic) • Oxycodone (Oxycontin, Roxicodone, others) • Tramadol (Ultram)
Sleep medications	• Flurazepam (Dalmane) • Temazepam (Restoril) • Triazolam (Halcion) • Zaleplon (Sonata) • Zolpidem (Ambien)

of the research points this way. But more recent reports suggest that it may be more of a two-way street, with nature and nurture each contributing their part to determine how well your mind ages.

This isn't surprising, considering that almost everything in life is a blend of nature and nurture. It seems to make sense that using your brain would keep it limber longer — but at the same time, diseases such as Alzheimer's don't always discriminate.

On a personal perspective, the key may be to focus on those factors that you have control over, just as you would with risk factors for heart disease or other illnesses. In employing strategies to enrich the life of your mind, you may very well be protecting and extending it as well.

Focus on solutions

Take a moment to consider the impact that your attitude may have on memory lapses. You may worry about a lapse and blame yourself. Or you cast it as a problem to be solved. Ask yourself how the problem may have developed. If you misplaced the car keys, maybe you were carrying them in a different coat pocket and forgot about them. If you lost a document at work, it could be because you were too busy trying to do three things at once.

Positive thinking leads to possible solutions: You resume carrying the keys in the same pocket you always have (and decide to keep a spare set on hand). Or you slow down on the job and pay more attention, especially when filing documents away.

The fact is, many people who claim to have trouble with memory actually don't. But they've developed such a poor attitude about their memory that they continually doubt themselves. They may know someone's name but are afraid to speak out for fear they might be wrong.

The alternative is to trust yourself. Instead of telling yourself, "I never remember names," substitute "That name will come back to me in a minute." Or, "I'm such a scatterbrain," can change to, "I sometimes forget, but I remember the things that are really important." Move from self-blame statements to positive messages.

Chapter 13

Research trends

Over the past few decades a massive worldwide effort has been made to investigate the causes of dementia and find ways to battle the disorder. Medical researchers are pursuing many leads on different fronts: risk factors, diagnosis, treatment of behavioral and cognitive symptoms, and prevention. Efforts are also directed toward improving caregiving strategies and providing more support options to caregivers.

This varied body of knowledge and resources grows at a rapid pace. Within the last five years alone, major advances have been made in identifying people at high risk for developing dementia. Many scientists agree that in the long run the prevention of Alzheimer's disease or delaying its onset may be as effective as — or even exceed — the results of any treatment strategy delivered after the disease process has started.

It would be difficult in this chapter to cover all of the ongoing dementia research, but some of the more prominent trends are highlighted. These trends involve research into causes of the disease, early diagnosis, treatment and prevention, and lifestyle factors. The last part of the chapter focuses on how individuals can participate in clinical trials that may provide some answers. The continued hope is that with new advances, there will soon be more effective means to prevent and treat dementia in all its forms.

Causes

Based on what current research suggests, it seems unlikely that a disease such as Alzheimer's is caused by a single factor. Instead, the common form of Alzheimer's that develops after age 65 is likely caused by the interactions of several factors, both genetic and environmental. Scientists working to unravel the mystery have identified several risk factors so far. In general, the presence of one risk factor isn't enough to cause the disease but, when combined with other risk factors, points the way to dementia.

In addition to establishing risk factors of dementia, researchers are also striving to better understand the underlying biological mechanisms that accompany the disease. Gaining a better perspective on what causes Alzheimer's makes it easier to develop treatment targeted for individual cases.

Following are some of the latest research findings that may reveal the potential causes of Alzheimer's disease. For more on the biological processes and risk factors associated with Alzheimer's, see Chapter 5.

Genetic risk factors

Some researchers are looking specifically at genetic factors that may put a person at greater risk of dementia. Although some genetic factors have been identified with the less common, inherited forms of Alzheimer's, such as the APP and presenilin genes, the APOE ε4 gene is of particular interest due to its association with the more common form of Alzheimer's. Another recently identified gene that may increase risk of Alzheimer's is known as the UBQLN1 gene.

APOE ε4. Increasingly, evidence confirms that APOE ε4, one of three common variants of the APOE gene, is a risk factor for both mild cognitive impairment and Alzheimer's. Experts still aren't sure about APOE's role in Alzheimer's disease but they have gained some clues about the natural biological functions of APOE. It appears that APOE is important in:

- Transport of cholesterol through the bloodstream
- Brain development and neuronal repair following injury
- Creation of synapses, the connection points between neurons

- Plasticity, or the capability of the brain to remodel itself in response to an injury
- Modifying inflammatory responses in the brain

It may be that weaknesses or abnormalities in any of these functions make a person more susceptible to cognitive decline and dementia. In particular, the ε4 variant may be more likely to be defective or have potentially toxic effects. For example, various studies have reported that people with the APOE ε4 variation have a greater number of amyloid beta deposits — a hallmark of Alzheimer's disease — than those with the APOE ε3 variation.

Because of growing evidence of APOE ε4's link to Alzheimer's, the gene variation has become a primary target for research. Scientists hope to better understand its biological role but also to develop treatments that might inhibit its damaging effects.

UBQLN1. Scientists may have pinpointed another genetic risk factor for Alzheimer's disease in variations of the UBQLN1 gene located on chromosome 9. Over the course of 10 years, researchers evaluated several families with histories of Alzheimer's disease in an effort to detect genetic risk factors for the disease. Their findings suggest that the UBQLN1 gene increases the risk for Alzheimer's disease, although perhaps not as much as APOE ε4. UBQLN1 appears to interact with the presenilin genes (PS1 and PS2) and may play a role in the degradation of proteins in the brain.

Aging and family history

Two commonly accepted risk factors for Alzheimer's disease are aging and family history. Generally, a person's risk of developing Alzheimer's increases with growing older, especially after age 65. Risk also increases if the person has close relatives who have Alzheimer's, and even more so if the relative with Alzheimer's developed the disease at an early age.

Some scientists speculate that, in fact, everyone is susceptible to Alzheimer's at some point in his or her lifetime, the only difference being the age at onset — something that might be a key genetic trait. For example, if a woman's father developed Alzheimer's at age 70, then she would inherit a tendency to develop Alzheimer's at around the same age.

To test their theory, these scientists collected the family histories of people with Alzheimer's, especially with regard to the age of onset. They also gathered information from older adults without dementia and their close relatives to serve as a reference. From this information, the research group worked to develop a schema that illustrated the pattern of Alzheimer's risk for older adults.

What they found was a more complex picture than previously believed. Although a relative's inherited risk does increase with age, it appears to peak at a certain time — close to the age at which their parent or sibling developed Alzheimer's — and then decline afterward, to a point where that person's risk is the same as someone who has no relatives with dementia. Also, the risk for close relatives decreases as the age of onset increases for the individual with Alzheimer's. The older a person is when he or she develops Alzheimer's, the lower the risk for his or her relatives.

What this may suggest is that as you age, genetic risk factors tend to become less important while environmental factors tend to become more influential.

Vascular risk factors

Evidence is mounting that factors such as chronic high blood pressure, elevated cholesterol or homocysteine levels, or a history of heart disease, heart attack or heart failure may increase a person's risk of Alzheimer's disease.

Scientists have yet to unravel the connections between vascular disease and dementia. But what they have discovered is that vascular cognitive impairment — the form of dementia that results from narrowed or blocked blood vessels in the brain— frequently develops at the same time as Alzheimer's disease. (For more information on vascular cognitive impairment, see Chapter 9.) In addition, the occurrence of the two forms of dementia together appears to intensify their signs and symptoms.

Tentative links have been made between high cholesterol and dementia, in part because the APOE ε4 gene variation is a risk factor for both cardiovascular disease and Alzheimer's disease. It's possible that the genetic programming for processing cholesterol in the body may also affect the onset of Alzheimer's.

Associations have also been observed between the risk factors for stroke, such as high blood pressure, and vascular cognitive impairment. High blood pressure can damage blood vessels in the brain leading to blockage or leakage of these vessels and insufficient blood flow to brain cells. Without necessary nutrients derived from the bloodstream, neurons will suffer damage and die.

Dementia has also been connected to elevated homocysteine levels. Homocysteine (ho-mo-SIS-te-un) is a naturally occurring amino acid in the body, used to make proteins and to maintain tissue. Elevated levels of homocysteine have been linked to a higher risk of cardiovascular disease. It may be that the risk for dementia actually is linked to a vitamin deficiency, because elevated levels of homocysteine can be due to low levels of folate, a type of vitamin B that helps to keep homocysteine from reaching toxic levels.

If cardiovascular factors do influence a person's risk of dementia, this raises the exciting possibility of prevention by managing diet and exercise and through medications, similar to what is currently prescribed for cardiovascular disease.

Underlying biological mechanisms

Many researchers are striving to understand exactly what processes occur in the brain that destroy its nerve cells and cause dementia. Two areas of research are prominent: the role of amyloid plaques and the role of neurofibrillary tangles.

Amyloid plaque formation. One theory regarding physiological changes in the brain that lead to Alzheimer's involves the aggregation of amyloid-beta protein fragments into long chains called amyloid fibrils, which in turn clump with other substances to form hard, insoluble plaques. These plaques appear in disproportionate numbers in the brains of people with Alzheimer's. For more information on the formation of amyloid plaques, see page 58.

Scientists continue to investigate how these plaques are formed and what role they play in the development of dementia. For example, a recent study examining the structure of amyloid fibrils found that they resemble molecular "zippers." In order for the fibrils to form, protein fragments must be lined up just right. When they do form, the fibrils zip up so tight that it's very difficult to undo them.

This may explain why plaques are so hard to get rid of. At the same time, this knowledge may lead to finding ways to disrupt fibril formation and potentially prevent the accumulation of plaques.

A missing link? A recent theory has emerged regarding a type of protein called amyloid-beta-derived diffusible ligands (ADDLs), miniscule toxic compounds that may precede the formation of amyloid plaques. Unlike the larger, more easily detected plaques, ADDLs are so small as to go undetected, even during a post-mortem examination. Some researchers believe that ADDLs may be the missing link between plaques and Alzheimer's disease.

Although people with Alzheimer's have a high number of plaques in their brains, many people with no dementia also have substantial amounts of plaques when their brains are examined during autopsy. The fact that a person can have plaques and not have Alzheimer's means the association between plaques and Alzheimer's may not be so direct. This calls into question the precise role of plaques in the disease process.

Through various studies and the examination of human brain cells, researchers have learned that ADDLs attack synapses, the points of contact between neurons. The loss of synapses disrupts the transfer of information from one cell to another, leading to communication breakdown. The researchers believe that this disruption is what causes the memory loss associated with Alzheimer's. What they also note is that the level of ADDLs is highly elevated in samples of brain tissue where Alzheimer's is present.

ADDLs may provide a new research target for diagnosis and therapy. For example, mice genetically programmed to develop plaques and tangles were vaccinated with antibodies to fight the plaques. Even though the amount of plaques the mice carried remained the same after vaccination, they showed an improvement in cognition including a rapid reversal of memory loss. Some scientists believe that the vaccine actually targeted ADDLs instead of the intended plaques and that's what led to the mice's recovery.

Scientists recently developed a test that can detect ADDLs in a person's cerebrospinal fluid, which hopefully will provide a way to better study the effect of ADDLs in people (see "Biomarkers and brain imaging techniques" on pages 205-208).

Neurofibrillary tangles. Abnormal masses of tau protein within the cell body — neurofibrillary tangles — are characteristic of several neurodegenerative disorders. Examples include Alzheimer's disease, frontotemporal dementia with parkinsonism (FTDP-17), corticobasal degeneration and progressive supranuclear palsy. For more information on neurofibrillary tangles, see page 59.

One current avenue of research is the role these neurofibrillary tangles play in dementia — are they a cause of the disease or a byproduct? To help answer this question, scientists are studying a type of mouse that exhibits these tau abnormalities. With this animal model, they can experiment with different medications that may be able to influence the formation of neurofibrillary tangles. If they find a medication that prevents or eliminates the tangles, this potentially may lead to a therapy helpful to humans.

Several aspects of these studies are worth noting. In certain disorders, the tangles are distributed in the brain in a pattern that's distinct from other disorders. Also, the tau protein's basic building blocks, amino acids, are sequenced differently in different dementias. Scientists are hoping to use these distribution patterns and the distinctive biochemical makeup of tau as "bar codes" to distinguish between different dementing disorders and help make a diagnosis.

Early diagnosis

Another trend of intense research lies in detecting dementia in its earliest stages. Because current drug therapies tend to be most helpful in early stages of the disease, diagnosing the disease as early as possible might allow for better response. Early detection also would allow doctors to target individuals for potentially preventive therapies or at least ones that delay the progression of dementia to its more severe stages.

As researchers work to identify signs and symptoms at the very early stages of Alzheimer's, they're also looking to develop tests that can help diagnose the disease at this stage. Some tests look for early cognitive or biological signs (markers) of dementia. Brain imaging techniques are also being explored for this purpose.

Precursor stage to dementia

Recently, researchers have made important advances in identifying a transitional stage between normal cognitive health and dementia. This stage is called mild cognitive impairment (for more information, see Chapter 11). Studies suggest that people with mild cognitive impairment (MCI) are not assured of getting dementia but nevertheless are at a high risk for developing the disease, particularly Alzheimer's — about 80 percent of people with the memory-related form of MCI go on to develop Alzheimer's.

People with MCI start forgetting things they normally would remember, and this begins to disrupt their daily activities. People around them notice the forgetfulness. However, the disruption is not to the degree of disability that's associated with dementia. Although everyone forgets things occasionally, people with MCI tend to develop a pattern of forgetfulness. Formal testing confirms that their memory function is low compared with others at their age and education level.

Because of its transitional nature, there are fine lines distinguishing MCI from normal and from dementia. Scientists are still working to establish a standard definition of MCI and uniform criteria for its diagnosis. Once these standards are determined, doctors will be able to diagnose MCI more accurately and, with more study, learn more about the causes of dementia.

Cognitive tests

Various interview-type tests — in which a person is required to answer a set of questions or accomplish a series of simple tasks — already exist that allow doctors to fairly accurately assess the cognitive status of a person being tested for dementia. Researchers are now looking to develop simple cognitive tests that could diagnose dementia in its earliest stage or accurately predict a person's risk of developing dementia several years down the line. This kind of testing would be particularly useful as new therapies are developed and become available.

Recently, a group of researchers set out to modify a standard test for dementia, which involves four separate recall tests based on a 10-word list. These tests consist of allowing a person to view a list of common words and then asking the person, either immediately or several minutes later, to recall as many words from memory as possible. Normally, a single score is used to determine whether cognitive impairment is present. But the researchers speculate that more information could be gleaned from the results if individual answers were weighted according to a technique called correspondence analysis. A modified version of the test increases the ability to detect mild cognitive impairment and early-stage dementia by about 12 percent.

A Canadian group of researchers found that a similar test was able to predict a person's 10-year risk of developing Alzheimer's with 70 percent accuracy. When this test was combined with two other tests — one testing a person's ability to recall animal names and the other a general information test — results were able to predict a person's five-year risk of Alzheimer's with even greater accuracy, over 80 percent. The researchers developed a fairly simple equation that factored in results of the three tests with age and years of education to determine the person's probability of developing Alzheimer's within five or 10 years.

Although other studies are needed to confirm usability of these tests, they may be useful in identifying high-risk individuals who would like to participate in clinical trials involving assessment or treatment for Alzheimer's.

Biomarkers and brain imaging techniques

Another aspect of early diagnosis is the identification of biological markers, substances found in the body that may signal an elevated risk of a condition or disease. Finding a biomarker for Alzheimer's disease would greatly facilitate doctors' ability to detect people at high risk and enable them to receive prompt treatment.

Some of the most characteristic features of dementia, for example, the plaques and tangles of Alzheimer's disease, are generally studied during autopsy after the person has died. Imaging techniques are now being developed that allow scientists to peer into the brains of people with dementia to help detect and monitor biomarkers and other changes that may be associated with the natural history of the disease. In addition, these imaging techniques will help scientists to monitor the brain's response to therapies, especially new, experimental ones.

Tracing amyloid beta. A group of scientists at Northwestern University have developed a type of stain called Pittsburgh Compound B (PIB) that readily sticks to the amyloid beta plaques that form in the living brain. (For more information on this new technique, see page 62 and Chapter 6.) The stain can be seen with the use of positron emission tomography (PET), a brain imaging technique that causes radioactive tracers, such as PIB, to light up on the imaging screen.

Previously, amyloid plaques could only be detected during autopsy. This new PIB compound, in conjunction with PET scanning, may allow physicians to quantify and monitor the amount of amyloid beta in a person's brain while they are living, and to learn more about the role of amyloid beta in Alzheimer's.

The compound was recently tested in humans for the first time by a group of researchers in Sweden. All study participants had donated their brain tissue for medical examination after death. The researchers found that images of the PIB stain followed much the same pattern as the plaques observed in postmortem studies of the participants' Alzheimer's-affected brains. These results confirm the ability of PIB to outline areas of amyloid beta deposition.

Although more trials need to be conducted before the compound might be considered for regular testing, it may help to answer the question of whether an increasing number of amyloid beta deposits are a part of normal aging or are a presymptomatic sign of Alzheimer's.

Detecting ADDLs. Other research has focused on detecting ADDLs, the toxic proteins mentioned earlier in the chapter that may be involved in the early stages of neuron degeneration. These potential Alzheimer's biomarkers have been very difficult to detect using available technology — individually, they measure a mere 5 nanometers wide (a nanometer is a millionth of a millimeter). Recently, however, scientists developed an ultrasensitive test that's able to measure the concentration of ADDLs in a person's cerebrospinal fluid, the fluid that surrounds, cushions and protects the brain and spinal cord.

A preliminary clinical trial found that healthy study participants showed a consistently lower level of ADDLs in their cerebrospinal fluid than participants diagnosed with Alzheimer's disease. The researchers noted that one person in particular, who was classified as healthy with no dementia, showed no significant amount of ADDLs but at the same time carried a moderate amount of plaques. This would seem to confirm the idea that ADDLs may be more closely associated with the disease process than plaques.

With the ability to measure the level of ADDLs in cerebrospinal fluid, scientists hope they'll be able to learn more about the role of these microscopic proteins in the development of Alzheimer's and possibly other forms of dementia. Scientists also hope to develop the test further so that it can be done with blood and urine samples, which are easier to obtain than cerebrospinal fluid.

Monitoring the hippocampus. The hippocampus is a brain structure that plays an essential role in a person's memory system. It's usually one of the first structures to be affected by Alzheimer's. The gradual loss of tissue associated with the disease results in visible shrinking (atrophy) of the hippocampus. To confirm a diagnosis of Alzheimer's, for example, doctors often use magnetic resonance imaging (MRI) to check for a smaller-than-normal volume of the hippocampal area (see pages 56-57).

But MRI measurements of the hippocampus are also being used for a number of other diagnostic and monitoring purposes:

Detecting mild cognitive impairment. Studies show that people with mild cognitive impairment (MCI) have a slightly smaller hippocampus than people who are cognitively normal (see page 179).

Predicting the progression of MCI to AD. People who have a small hippocampus at the time MCI is diagnosed progress to Alzheimer's faster than those who have a larger hippocampus.

Monitoring the progression of dementia. A series of MRI scans can reveal the rate at which a person's hippocampus is shrinking. This rate correlates with levels of neuron loss elsewhere in the brain and cognitive impairment associated with dementia. For example, the rate of atrophy in people with MCI is higher than in normal adults, and is also higher in those with MCI who eventually progress to AD than in those whose MCI remains stable.

Monitoring the effectiveness of experimental therapies.
Although no studies have yet confirmed the ability of MRIs to
reveal the effects of an experimental drug on hippocampal atrophy
— whether the therapy is successful in stopping or slowing the rate
of neuron loss — the possibility does exist.

Other magnetic resonance tests are being explored for use as
diagnostic and monitoring tools. Magnetic resonance spectroscopy
is a test used to measure the amounts of certain metabolic substances (metabolites) in the body. Some studies have found that
abnormal levels of certain metabolites may indicate the degree of
Alzheimer's progression.

Diffusion-weighted MRI is another way to measure atrophy of
the hippocampus. The test can measure microscopic structural
changes by measuring the mobility of water molecules in the brain.
If the hippocampus is even microscopically smaller than normal,
for example, water molecules will have more room to move around
than in a brain whose hippocampus fills more space. The technical
term for this measurement is "apparent diffusion coefficient." A
person with MCI who is progressing to AD is likely to have a higher apparent diffusion coefficient than one who is not.

Now that positron emission tomography (PET) has been used to
view amyloid plaques in the living brain, scientists are hoping to
do the same using MRI, which is a more common and less expensive procedure. To do so, scientists are working on creating a special contrast agent that can cross the brain's protective barrier
(blood-brain barrier) and bind directly with the plaques so that the
plaques can be seen on an MRI scan.

Measuring the activity of the brain

Another way of detecting differences between a brain that is cognitively normal and one that has cognitive impairment is by measuring not the volume of brain structures but their level of activity.

All brain cells use blood sugar (glucose) for energy during normal cellular operations. PET scans can measure the metabolism
(chemical processing) of glucose in the brain, as well as other vital
functions such as blood flow and oxygen use. Studies of people
with Alzheimer's and MCI using PET technology show that these

individuals have areas of reduced glucose metabolism, meaning there's less cellular activity.

A similar form of brain imaging called single photon emission computed tomography (SPECT) is capable of measuring blood flow. It also has been used to show reduced brain activity in people with dementia. The information revealed on SPECT images correlates well with the results of cognitive tests, suggesting that the physiological changes captured on the images reflect the development of cognitive deficits.

Both of the PET and SPECT tests may be used to help confirm a diagnosis of dementia, but researchers are hoping the scans will help identify individuals at risk of dementia, before symptoms become evident and severe damage to brain cells has occurred. PET and SPECT also have been used to predict which individuals with MCI progress to Alzheimer's and which remain stable.

Functional MRI (fMRI) is another imaging test that measures neuron activity in the brain. When asked to perform different tasks, people with MCI and AD show different patterns of activity than people who are cognitively normal. More long-term studies are needed to see if fMRI can detect memory impairment before it becomes symptomatic.

If a disease-modifying drug becomes available, these and other imaging tests may help evaluate the effectiveness of such a drug.

Treatment and prevention

Currently, treatment of Alzheimer's disease includes medications that try to stabilize cognitive function, if only for a short period of time. Drugs approved by the Food and Drug Administration (FDA) include cholinesterase inhibitors — donepezil (Aricept), galantamine (Razadyne) and rivastigmine (Exelon), used mostly during the mild and moderate stages of AD — and most recently memantine (Namenda), a drug aimed at improving late-stage symptoms. (For more information on these drugs, see Chapter 6.)

It may be that a disease such as Alzheimer's begins decades before a person experiences signs and symptoms. Increasingly, even as investigators work to diagnose the disease at its earliest stage, they're also looking to arrest its progress when the effects may still be reversible or even prevented. Currently, several strategies are being closely studied.

Alzheimer's vaccine

Several years ago, when researchers were able to show that a vaccine injected into cognitively impaired mice was able to reduce deposits of amyloid plaque and improve memory loss, it generated excitement about the possibility of an anti-Alzheimer's vaccine in humans. Investigators began preliminary studies of the AN1792 vaccine in humans, but these trials eventually were halted because some participants developed brain inflammation as a side effect.

Scientists haven't lost hope, however, and continue to work on second-generation vaccines that may not produce such dangerous side effects. In addition, researchers continue to follow certain participants of the original study who didn't develop brain inflammation. They've found that these participants did better on neurological testing than participants who had received placebos.

Immunized participants also showed a reduced amount of plaques in the brain and decreased levels of tau protein — the protein that's involved in the formation of tangles — in cerebrospinal fluid. These are all positive signs and, if side effects can be minimized, immunization may yet prove to be an effective therapy.

Secretase inhibitors

In Chapter 5, you learned about the amyloid-clipping enzymes (proteases) and how they're involved in the formation of plaques. Scientists believe that if they can create a drug that inhibits the actions of these proteases, it will decrease the number of plaques that are formed and thus the degeneration of neurons.

Scientists face several challenges in this area of research. For one, the drug must be able to cross the blood-brain barrier that surrounds and protects the brain from foreign substances in the blood. This barrier maintains a safe and stable environment for the brain and spinal cord and generally doesn't allow molecules that are too large or too highly charged to pass through.

Also, the drug must be selective enough to target only the harmful actions of these enzymes and not interfere with their normal functions in the body.

This is a tall order, but various groups of researchers are working to understand these enzymes better and find a therapeutic counteraction to their involvement in Alzheimer's disease.

Cardiovascular therapies

Some studies of statins — cholesterol-lowering drugs — have indicated that regular use of these medications in mid-life decreases a person's risk of dementia. This not only appears to confirm a link between high cholesterol and an increased risk for Alzheimer's disease, but also offers the possibility of reducing a person's risk for dementia by controlling cholesterol levels through diet and medication. The theory is still controversial, however, as other studies have failed to find a similar association.

Another large study found that people who took medications to lower blood pressure had a reduced risk of vascular dementia. Because vascular dementia and Alzheimer's increasingly appear connected, controlling high blood pressure may have a therapeutic effect on Alzheimer's, as well.

Homocysteine levels in the blood can be reduced by consuming more folic acid and vitamins B6 and B12. If elevated homocysteine is determined to be a risk factor for dementia, increased dietary intake of these nutrients may be a way to prevent the disease. But several long-term trials are necessary to test this theory before it can be prescribed as a preventive measure against dementia.

Antioxidants

Researchers have been studying whether antioxidants such as vitamin E may protect against the progression of Alzheimer's. But research published in April 2005 in the *New England Journal of Medicine* indicates no benefit from taking vitamin E. The research showed no significant difference in the progression from mild cognitive impairment to Alzheimer's disease in a group of people taking vitamin E compared with a control group not taking vitamin E. (For more details on the study, see Chapter 11.)

Scientists continue to investigate the potential risks and benefits of vitamin E for Alzheimer's. A single trial using high doses of vitamin E as therapy for moderate stages of Alzheimer's appeared to be beneficial. Results from another study suggest that food sources of vitamin E, such as vegetable oils and seed oils, may be more protective than supplements of vitamin E. Other researchers, examining multiple studies of vitamin E, point out that high doses of vitamin E (more than 400 IU a day) may actually be harmful to some people, although this was not demonstrated in the moderate-stage Alzheimer's trial.

Anti-inflammatory agents

Several studies indicate that the NSAIDs ibuprofen (Advil, Motrin, others), naproxen sodium (Aleve) and indomethacin (Indocin) may reduce the risk of developing Alzheimer's disease. As described in Chapter 5, inflammation may play a role in the Alzheimer's disease process. What isn't known is whether the inflammation is a cause or simply an effect of the disease.

In late 2004, investigators halted a major trial studying the effects of naproxen and celecoxib (Celebrex), another anti-inflammatory drug, in Alzheimer's disease. The stoppage occurred because findings from another unrelated cancer study involving celecoxib suggested that the drug might increase a person's risk of heart disease. Although the Alzheimer's trial was halted, investigators nonetheless are continuing to examine existing data from the study, which had started in 2001.

The Alzheimer's trial and the cancer trial were the first long-term studies to test these kinds of drugs for uses other than for what they're currently approved. Because NSAIDs also can cause serious gastrointestinal bleeding, more conclusive clinical trials need to be completed before it's clear whether people should take NSAIDs solely to prevent Alzheimer's.

Estrogen

Early studies suggest that estrogen may have a protective effect against Alzheimer's, but more recent studies involving women who already had AD have failed to confirm this positive effect.

In fact, results from a large-scale study called the Women's Health Initiative Memory Study indicated an increased risk of dementia for women 65 years and older who had taken hormone replacement therapy — either estrogen alone or a combination of estrogen and progestin. This study had several limitations that reduced its applicability to all women. For example, it didn't study the effect of estrogen on the risk of dementia if given to women younger than 65. Nevertheless, it provided no support for, and even indicated against the use of, hormone replacement therapy to protect against cognitive decline in women over the age of 65.

Other studies showed more positive results. They suggest that early hormone therapy — given usually when a woman is in her 50s to treat menopausal symptoms — may have cognitive benefits. Some researchers speculate that this early therapy may have protective effects while later use becomes harmful.

Recently, a study designed to evaluate the effects of raloxifene (Evista), a selective estrogen-receptor modulator (SERM), on postmenopausal women with osteoporosis, found that participants receiving a higher dosage of the drug had a reduced risk of mild cognitive impairment. Raloxifene isn't a hormone like estrogen but it mimics some of estrogen's effects. It may be that the drug provides cognitive benefits while avoiding other harmful effects. For example, unlike estrogen, raloxifene isn't associated with an increased risk of stroke or other cardiovascular events. The study's results are tentative, and additional studies are needed to confirm this potentially therapeutic role for raloxifene.

Lifestyle factors

Some studies point toward the importance of healthy living, intellectual stimulation and social relationships in preventing cognitive decline. For example, some researchers believe that lifelong mental exercise and learning may promote the growth of additional synapses, the connections between neurons, and delay the onset of dementia. Other researchers argue that advanced education simply gives a person more experience with the types of memory and thinking involved in tests used to measure dementia. This may provide some people with a cognitive "reserve" that compensates for other cognitive deficits.

Evidence also suggests that being physically fit and staying connected with others maintains cognitive performance and reduces a person's risk of dementia. Read Chapter 12, "Staying Mentally Sharp," to learn more about things that you can do that may help you keep your brain healthy and active.

How to participate in a clinical trial

It's difficult, if not impossible, for scientists to conduct research without volunteer participants. This is where the public can play a vital part in the pursuit of better treatment and prevention of dementia. Nevertheless, a decision to enroll in a clinical trial should be considered carefully. In the case of Alzheimer's disease, this decision often rests with the entire family, rather than just one person. To help families with this decision, the Alzheimer's Association has prepared the following list of considerations to take into account:

- Along with your physician, explore whether it's in your loved one's best interest to become involved.
- Be prepared to answer questions about your loved one's condition.
- Expect further screening by the study site to determine eligibility for the trial. Only a minority of interested people may qualify for a particular trial.
- Be aware of the time commitment and other responsibilities involved in participating, such as making trips to the study site, administering the drug and reporting health-related changes to the study coordinators.
- Understand that clinical studies may involve some risk, as they determine the effectiveness and safety of a drug. By the time a drug reaches testing in humans, however, researchers are fairly optimistic of obtaining positive results with few side effects.

Keeping it all in perspective

There's so much research surrounding Alzheimer's disease and dementia that it may seem bewildering at times. And not that infrequently, study results appear to contradict each other, leaving most people wondering whether these "advances" will ever truly help them or their loved ones.

New therapies take time to develop and even then, many additional studies must be done to support the initial findings before

- Know that not all participants are given the treatment being tested. In almost every study, there's a group that receives a placebo, or inactive substance, and a group that receives the experimental treatment. This allows researchers to compare the two groups.
- Realize that individuals receiving the placebo are just as important as those receiving the treatment. Clinical drug trials can't be completed without a control group. If the drug yields positive results, the participants who have been given the placebo may now be given the option of receiving the experimental drug.
- Always remember to ask questions. Researchers should be able to answer your questions satisfactorily. If you feel uncomfortable at any point, you always have the option of not continuing with the study.

To find out more about clinical trials for Alzheimer's disease, you can look up one of the following Internet addresses:

- Alzheimer's Association: Clinical trials *www.alz.org/research/clintrials/*
- National Institute on Aging: Alzheimer's Disease Clinical Trials Database *www.alzheimers.org/trials/basicsearch.html*
- National Institutes of Health: Database of all clinical trials *www.clinicaltrials.gov*

safety and effectiveness can be confirmed. Some people may feel that even though so much is being discovered, it won't be soon enough to be of any use to them or their loved ones. But people whose lives are affected by a neurodegenerative disease have the opportunity to further research by participating in ongoing clinical trials. In addition, volunteers who participate in clinical trials are eligible to receive either state-of-the-art therapy or a potentially helpful experimental therapy.

Most researchers expect to see major progress in the treatment and prevention of Alzheimer's in the next few decades. And in this, we can only hope that they are right.

Action guide

for caregivers

The structure of this action guide represents, in very general terms, the pathway that caregivers might follow on their journey with a loved one through the disease process of dementia. Tips and strategies from the various sections can be read all at once, or you may choose to focus only on the most relevant sections at a given time. As the dementia progresses, you'll likely interpret and adapt this content in new and different ways. The more understanding you have of the disease and the caregiving journey, the better you're able to cope with today, tomorrow and the years ahead.

Sections

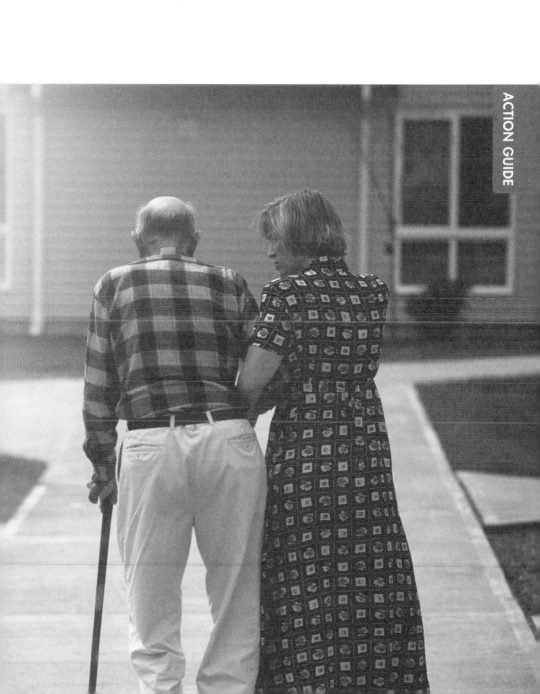

Receiving a diagnosis

You've just learned from the doctor that a loved one — parent, sibling or friend — is diagnosed in the early stages of Alzheimer's disease. You may have been hoping to hear that the forgetfulness and confusion was simply due to aging, or that the symptoms would disappear with a medication adjustment. You're flooded with disbelief. It's hard to imagine something like this happening to someone so close to you.

It probably was difficult to acknowledge your growing concerns about a loved one, and then to bring those concerns to the doctor's attention. Because the onset of dementia is often gradual, symptoms could be passed off as part of growing old. And the word *dementia* is associated with some of your worst fears: Untreatable and unrelenting, loss of self-identity and awareness, total dependence on others.

These are strong emotions and sensitivities to work through. Your loved one may not have agreed that something was wrong or may have resisted the doctor visit. But now you and your loved one must face the consequences of the diagnosis together.

Coming to terms

Family members often play a key role in the diagnosis of dementia for a loved one. They're generally the ones who first notice how memory loss, disorientation and mood swings are disrupting a person's life. They also may be the ones receiving the brunt of those changes. Family members often initiate the first doctor visit to find out if something's wrong.

There's generally a two- to three-year delay from the time family members begin to notice symptoms to the time that they schedule the evaluation. The delay may be due to confusion about what's considered normal age-related memory changes versus more serious developments. However, the delay may simply be part of the process — a gradual realization that the changes in your loved one aren't getting better and may be due to dementia.

Denial is often the earliest and strongest emotion that family members feel. It's a normal response to the situation — as family members accept the reality of a progressive, incurable disorder in a loved one, the more distrust they have of the future and their ability to cope. Denial provides a protective buffer from uncertainty.

Sometimes, instead of denial, family members experience anger. People who feel anger are expressing the perceived unfairness of the illness: "Why us, why now?" They're considering the losses that the illness brings to future plans. Emotions such as fear and anxiety are commonly mixed in.

In some situations, a diagnosis of dementia brings a sense of relief. Family members can understand why their loved one's memory has been so unreliable, and they can make sense of other changes that have occurred.

The journey from denial to acceptance isn't a linear path. Family members, and even the person receiving the diagnosis of dementia, find themselves at different stages at different times. At times, you may feel like you're the only one in this situation, but you're never alone. Millions of people in the United States and around the world have Alzheimer's disease or other forms of dementia. Everyone works through their feelings and adjusts emotionally at their own pace.

In the past, it may have seemed pointless to get a diagnosis of dementia. There was little that could be done to prevent or treat a disorder like Alzheimer's disease. But that's no longer the case. Medications for dementia are most effective when started early.

Range of emotions

A diagnosis of Alzheimer's disease or other form of dementia can cause you to feel any of the following moods and emotions:

- Disbelief
- Shock
- Fear
- Relief
- Embarrassment
- Confusion
- Anger
- Sadness
- Devastation
- Loss
- Numbness

Early symptoms of dementia

People seek an evaluation for dementia primarily because changes in behavior or mental function are noticeably disrupting their lives. Listed below are some of the most common symptoms of the early stages of dementia. Because every individual is so different and the causes of dementia are so varied, most people don't experience all of these symptoms — and the symptoms develop in different ways.

Memory loss. A person with dementia will frequently forget things, often recent events.

Difficulty performing familiar tasks. A person with dementia will have problems completing tasks he or she may have done many times before, such as following a recipe, using an appliance or performing a job-related task.

Problems with language. A person with dementia often forgets simple words or substitutes the wrong word, making communication difficult.

Disorientation to time and place. A person with dementia may become lost in familiar places and unable to get back home.

Poor or decreased judgment. A person with dementia may buy items he or she doesn't need or spend large sums of money irresponsibly.

Problems with abstract thinking. A person with dementia may forget what the numbers in a checkbook represent or what needs to be done with them.

Misplacing things. A person with dementia may misplace things in unusual places such as putting an iron in the refrigerator or a wristwatch in the sugar bowl.

Changes in mood or behavior. A person with dementia may experience unusually strong mood swings for no apparent reason, or behave inappropriately.

Changes in personality. A person with dementia may seem different from his or her usual self in ways that are difficult to pinpoint: suspicious, irritable, anxious or short tempered.

Loss of initiative. A person with dementia may become passive and withdrawn, sleeping more than usual and sitting in front of the television for hours.

Informing your loved one

There are no guidelines for what to say to a person who has been diagnosed with dementia. Certain factors are important to consider, such as how advanced the dementia symptoms are or how well the person comprehends what's being said. In most cases, telling the truth should be the usual practice.

The Alzheimer's Association believes that people have a moral and legal right to know their diagnosis if they have the capacity to understand it. Among individuals with more advanced stages of the disease, an explanation of their diagnosis may have little value, particularly if they've lost the ability to comprehend. But among individuals in the early stages of Alzheimer's disease, informing them of their diagnosis allows them to take a more active role in planning their future. With knowledge of the diagnosis, a person in the early stages of dementia can still:

- Plan life experiences that give them comfort and pleasure
- Prepare legal documents that specify how they'll be cared for in advanced stages of the disease
- Consider enrolling in research programs and clinical trials
- Participate in dementia-related support groups
- Participate in drug therapy that's generally effective in early stages of the disease

Health care professionals and family members have struggled over how to break the news about a diagnosis, only to have the individual respond, "That's what I've felt all along." People diagnosed with Alzheimer's disease may actually feel a sense of relief because the diagnosis explains the cause of their concern.

Some individuals, however, express disbelief and question what the doctor is telling them. You may want to describe the diagnosis as a problem with memory rather than using words such as *dementia* or *Alzheimer's disease.*

Your overall goal is to provide information about the diagnosis in a considerate and sensitive way that's appropriate for your loved one and that avoids unnecessary despair. If family members feel that their words and actions are in the best interest of the person with the disease, then they've likely chosen the best approach.

ACTION GUIDE

First person: Is knowing necessary?

A doctor has just diagnosed my elderly mother with Alzheimer's disease. Her short-term memory is already impaired. Should I tell her about the diagnosis? If so, how much should I tell her?

In deciding whether to tell your mother that she has Alzheimer's disease, consider the effect that this information may have on her general disposition. Does your mother recognize that she has memory problems? If she's often frustrated by her inability to remember things and calls herself dumb or stupid, knowledge of the diagnosis may help to remind her that the problems are due to the disease. You can say, "Mom, you're not stupid, you have Alzheimer's disease." This may reduce self-blame and negative moods.

On the other hand, if your mother doesn't realize that she has memory problems, trying to convince her that she has Alzheimer's may only frustrate the both of you. You may choose not to say anything. Some caregivers feel distress about keeping secrets and withholding information. Other caregivers feel that telling will only upset their loved ones. It's OK to do what feels right to you.

If you do decide to tell your mother, she may not respond in a way that you might expect. Alzheimer's makes people forget they have the condition — so you may have to tell your mother more than once. Keep in mind that the disease may impair your mother's ability to fully grasp the diagnosis. Many people, hearing for the first time they have Alzheimer's, appear to make no response at all. Don't be surprised if this is the case with your mother.

If you decide not to tell your mother, it still may help to talk about her memory problems — instead of ignoring them. For example, you can say, "Mom, we bought a weekly pill organizer to help you keep track of your medicines. This will make life easier and help with your memory problems."

Telling others about the diagnosis

Caregivers often wonder whom to tell about the diagnosis and when to tell them. This can be a frightening time for your loved one — he or she may not want to feel "under the microscope," with people closely watching for signs of illness. You may be torn between protecting your loved one's privacy and sharing something of the emotional rollercoaster you're on. Consider the following suggestions:

- Start the process by creating a list of those people who could most likely support you if informed of the diagnosis. A strong support network is a valuable resource for caregivers.
- Notifying neighbors may be particularly important. They're likely to contact you or offer assistance if they notice unusual behavior on the part of your loved one or if your loved one seems to be wandering and confused.
- Send letters providing details of the diagnosis and signs and symptoms that your loved one is experiencing. Describe how the disease will progress and may affect your lives in the future.
- Often, the more specific you can be about your needs, the more likely people can provide help. For example, rather than hinting that you're uncomfortable driving across town in traffic, you might say, "We're looking for help getting to doctor appointments (and here are the scheduled times)." Rather than complaining that lifting and bending bothers you or that you don't trust leaving your loved one in the house alone, you might say, "Can you help once a week with yard work?"
- Be sure to express your own needs as well as those of your loved one. Even if your loved one can no longer directly engage in conversation, you may appreciate visitors who provide emotional support or hands-on assistance.
- Consider sending a written update every three to six months to keep friends and family aware of you and your loved one's condition. Your local Alzheimer's Association chapter can provide information about the disease process that you might include.

Explaining the disease to children

Adults may choose to shield young children from the knowledge that a relative has dementia. But children often recognize when something is wrong. Your loved one's behavior may seem frightening or disturbing to them, especially if the children don't understand why that behavior is occurring. Here are ways to help you support young children during this time of uncertainty:

- Try to share information in simple terms that children can understand. Focus on behavioral symptoms and not on the science of the disease. This will help children cope better with the personality changes they'll observe.
- Children may feel scared, confused, embarrassed, angry, sad, or guilty about what's happening. Reassure them that it's no one's fault — not the person's fault and not the children's fault. Your loved one can't help the way he or she is acting.
- Children often ask blunt questions: Will I get this disease? Is Grandma crazy? What will happen next? Try to answer the questions honestly and with as much reassurance as possible.
- Draw out worries and concerns by asking the children about changes they've observed in your loved one. Help them imagine what it would be like to have the disease.
- Prepare the children for later changes that may occur, such as language problems, challenging behaviors and the inability to perform routine tasks.
- Watch for signs of withdrawal, poor school performance, headaches, stomachaches or other minor ailments in the children. This may signal that they're having difficulty coping.
- Suggest ways to help children to interact with your loved one: "Grandma has a hard time understanding us, so we need to be gentle and speak slowly to her."
- Provide activities that the children and your loved one can enjoy together, such as looking at a photo album, listening to music or doing a simple crafts project.
- Use books and videos to enrich your discussion with the children. The local Alzheimer's Association chapter may be a source of these materials.

Leaving employment

Some people in the early stages of dementia are able to continue working for awhile. But soon, they'll need to leave their jobs. Ending a career can be a painful process. The following may help your loved one through this transition with dignity.

- Inform an employer soon after your loved one receives the diagnosis. Ask whether work tasks may be simplified or work hours decreased. It may be easier to phase out employment rather than quit abruptly.
- Dementia affects judgment, reaction time and problem-solving skills. Consider whether the job requires decisions that could jeopardize the safety of your loved one or others. See if it's possible for your loved one to be reassigned to easier tasks.
- Your loved one may have mixed feelings about telling co-workers. Offer to be with your loved one at the time and, if appropriate, keep co-workers informed of new developments.
- A consistent routine may help your loved one continue to function without relying heavily on memory skills.
- Not being able to work may hasten the loss of self-identity. Reassure your loved one and bolster his or her sense of accomplishment. You can compile a scrapbook with highlights of his or her work life, with pictures, mementos and notes from colleagues.
- Look for activities that he or she can still participate in. Ask your loved one for help with household tasks.
- It may be helpful to maintain the regular hours of a work routine. For example, if your loved one previously went to the office at 8 a.m., you might leave the house together around that time and go for a cup of coffee.
- Your loved one may be able to attend elder care programs during regular work hours. Many caregivers find it helpful to describe this time as "going to work."
- Watch for signs of depression as work skills deteriorate. These signs include changes in appetite and sleep patterns. Other characteristic signs are excessive crying and anger.

Becoming a caregiver

Your spouse or parent has just been diagnosed with Alzheimer's disease. You have many questions and concerns about what to do next. The doctor may have given you good information and referred you to local resources that provide support. But it will take time to assimilate the news.

Often, it's not clear exactly when caregivers become caregivers. Maybe you feel like you've been in a caregiving role for some time already. Or maybe you never thought of yourself as a caregiver before — and, even now, you're not sure if you can become one.

It may be that you assumed the caregiver role as soon as you noticed the first symptoms. This may have occurred even if you weren't prepared to believe that the changes were anything more than normal aging. Perhaps your father could no longer pay his bills or keep track of medications. Maybe he needed help getting dressed or working a coffee maker. It may have seemed like very little help at the time — but that one step quickly turned into more and more responsibilities.

Alternatively, you may have identified yourself as a caregiver recently, at the moment the diagnosis was made. At last you're able to put a label on the changes that you've witnessed over the past months and this may have triggered your desire to assume a caregiving role.

In fact, the point at which people feel they've become caregivers varies with each situation and within each relationship. The realization forms at its own pace. It may be a conscious decision or it may just seem to happen. But however your decision came about, what's important is that you're working to meet your loved one's needs and best interests.

What is a caregiver?

A caregiver is anyone who takes responsibility for the basic needs of another person, either temporarily or permanently. This may include physical care and guidance as well as companionship and emotional support. The caregiver may be required to make important decisions regarding treatment, enlist medical services and represent a loved one's interests legally and financially. There are many mundane chores involved such as housecleaning, laundry, yard work, errand running and chauffeuring. At the same time, a caregiver must tend to his or her own mental and physical health. There also may be a career and family to maintain.

Caregivers can't control the course that dementia takes but they can shape the manner in which they support and care for their loved ones. Caregivers also can strengthen their abilities to cope with the additional, unrelenting, all-consuming responsibilities they've assumed. You can expect to play a very active role in the lives you and your loved one will lead in the months ahead.

Start by increasing your knowledge. The more you understand about how dementia will affect your loved one, the better you'll be able to guide him or her through the disease process and make a positive impact. The disease-related changes will seem less mysterious to you, and you may find it easier to adapt your care to them.

It's also important to have realistic expectations of what care you can or cannot provide. You'll likely be the central person in your loved one's life. You can provide high-quality care, but you also need to be ready to adjust, willing to acknowledge limitations and expect a few missteps.

In the early stages of dementia, your loved one still may be able to perform simple tasks with little supervision. But there are some functions — such as managing money and driving a car — that, even at early stages of the disease, are no longer possible without serious risk. At some point, sooner rather than later, your loved one will need to stop or be eased out of these responsibilities.

ACTION GUIDE

Stages of dementia

The signs and symptoms of dementia are described in Chapter 1 of this book. As the dementia progresses, your loved one's physical and emotional status may be gauged by the changing demands placed on the caregiver. Following may give you some idea of what to expect through the course of the disease:

Mild stage. Individuals in a mild stage of dementia will function best in familiar locations, such as at home, and by following well-organized schedules. They can manage many personal-care needs and home responsibilities, generally with minimal supervision. Simple written reminders and memory aids may help this process. They're aware of simple errors or digressions and able to correct them. They're able to learn new tasks when some instruction is provided. They benefit from home health services and daily checks. They're able to do limited travel outside the home.

Moderate stage. Individuals in a moderate stage of dementia will function best with consistent, predictable routines and when minimal expectations placed on them. They're able to feed themselves and perform simple tasks of personal care. Attention span is short — generally no more than one to three minutes. Visual cues are often needed for them to start tasks and then to continue performing them. Mood changes and emotional swings are common occurrences. Background noise and visual stimulation should be kept to a minimum because individuals with dementia generally aren't able to mask out these distractions. Safety becomes a primary concern. They're able to walk but will tend to wander away and be unable to avoid objects in their paths.

Severe stage. Individuals in a severe stage of dementia will need assistance with the activities of daily living, including feeding, bathing and toileting. They may be able to sit in a supported chair for brief periods and to feed self with hand-over-hand assistance. They can hold objects placed in the hand and move body parts in response to gentle stimuli. Their gaze can follow visual contrast and bright colors, and they'll respond to familiar music and sounds. Be in their field of vision before touching them to avoid startling. Gentle massage may calm them if they become agitated.

Changing roles and responsibilities

When a loved one experiences the impairment of memory and executive skills, a caregiver will become responsible for making decisions, organizing affairs and managing a schedule for that person. When this inevitable transition occurs, you may recognize a profound change in the familiar roles that had existed previously between yourself and your loved one.

Roles are distinct from responsibilities, which are the jobs people do. Roles refer to positions that someone assumes within the family, be it as parent, spouse, homemaker, decision-maker or advice-giver. Roles are established over many years, making them a little more difficult to transfer from a loved one to you.

Different roles and responsibilities don't mean the end to a relationship, only that it will change. You may be put in a role that, previously, your loved one had taken particular pride in. Spouses often feel uncomfortable about assuming responsibilities once held by their partners. You may struggle to balance the checkbook or cook a meal if that hadn't been your responsibility before.

You may become responsible for functions that your loved one considers personal and private. At some point, you may have to limit or remove something that your loved one holds dear. Children often hesitate to decide personal matters for a parent, for example, moving from a private home to assisted-living quarters.

These changes require emotional adjustments. As awkward and uncomfortable as you may feel, you must come to terms with the fact that people with dementia, even at an early stage of the disease, will need someone to step in and help them with certain tasks and with certain decisions. Even if your loved one seems resentful or angry with your help, you're responding to the demands that the disease has placed on both of you.

The process of accepting and adapting to new roles and responsibilities will take on many new dimensions, depending on the manner in which the relationship may have functioned in the past. Over time, this process can be a profoundly positive experience. For some caregivers, it unearths unknown reserves of resilience, patience, and compassion.

ACTION GUIDE

Adjusting your expectations

As your loved one experiences the changes brought on by dementia, he or she will require increasing amounts of assistance from you. You may ultimately be "on call" for your loved one 24 hours a day, seven days a week. The activities of daily living, along with housecleaning, shopping, paying bills and providing transportation, eventually will become your full responsibility. You also may become the primary emotional support for your loved one, who will be watching you for cues that indicate how to react or what to do next. Along with keeping your own life on course, that's a lot for one person to manage!

Having realistic expectations of your loved one's capabilities makes the experience easier. Be aware of what tasks the person should still be able to perform and what may be too difficult, frustrating or complex. Expect that the confusion and attention impairment brought on by dementia can disrupt simple routines on one day but not the next.

For example, imagine that your loved one becomes confused and puts shoes on the wrong feet. If you respond by saying, "What are you doing? You've put your shoes on wrong!" your loved one may become frightened and withdraw. You can frame your response in a way that your loved one can understand and not feel threatened by. For example, gently explain that you'd like to see the shoes so that you can polish them — then help put them on the correct feet. This helps make the experience positive.

You can't hope to protect your loved one from hurt feelings in every situation. And each day may take a slightly different turn. There will be moments of misunderstanding and tension. Try to view these moments in the context of your expectations.

Of course, realistic expectations also apply to you, the caregiver. A daily schedule and to-do list are good to follow, but with all the uncertainties and vagaries of the disease, you cannot expect to accomplish everything or rush the process or make up time. Learning from your experience can help you prepare for future changes, which in turn may make it a bit easier to guide your loved one through this journey.

First person: Adjusting to a new relationship

On a visit, Sarah noticed her mother, Lucy, wearing dirty clothes. She also found three weeks worth of unopened mail in a laundry basket. Sarah suspected something was wrong because her mom was always meticulous and organized. After a complete medical evaluation, Lucy was diagnosed with Alzheimer's disease. Sarah decided to move in with her mother. However, as Sarah became more involved in her mother's care, Lucy became agitated and sometimes angry with her.

When people with dementia become frustrated or scared, they often become angry. Other factors may combine to make the reaction more extreme — a reaction termed *catastrophic*. This may be due to being quizzed, feeling insecure or ignored, being made to feel like a child, feeling embarrassed, being reprimanded, or reacting to a tense situation. There are things you can do to limit agitation.

Make sure your loved one gets enough sleep. Fatigue can increase agitation.

Don't expect too much. Tasks that a loved one could do months ago may be too difficult now. Adapt the tasks as necessary.

Establish a routine. Routine can provide a sense of purpose and accomplishment.

Don't argue with or quiz your loved one. If you need to ask questions, make them clear and easy to understand.

Keep the environment simple and consistent. Changes — even small ones — can cause agitation.

Try not to show feelings of irritation or impatience. Respond to your loved one in a calm manner.

Provide understanding. Say, "I'm sorry this is so difficult right now" or reassure with a hug or back rub.

Take the blame. If your loved one blames you for something, recognize this as part of the disease. Don't argue.

Don't respond with physical force. Consider the five Rs: remain calm, respond to feelings, reassure the person, remove yourself, return later.

Consult a doctor. Agitation can be aggravated by physical symptoms of pain, discomfort, physical illness or depression.

Impact on career

Young adults or spouses caring for someone with an early-onset form of dementia may need to negotiate around the demands of a career. You may feel torn between wanting to focus on your loved one and attending to your job. Even if you have satisfactory care arrangements during work hours, if your loved one is restless at night, you'll suffer from sleep deprivation.

- Some caregivers are able to set up an alternate work schedule with their employer by cutting back on hours, job sharing or taking a leave of absence.
- While on the job, you may worry continually about your loved one. Consider all of the resources that your community might offer to help care for your loved one while you work.
- If you're thinking of leaving your job, consider the ramifications of this action. Quitting your job may include the loss of income, benefits and security, as well as losing your sense of identity. However, staying with your job may be difficult if you can't arrange alternate care.

Before making a final decision, take *your* needs into account. Many full-time caregivers have found themselves more stressed and at odds with their loved ones than before they left their jobs. Placing your loved one in an care facility may be a better solution.

Long-distance support

Even if you live far away, your support can be critical to a primary caregiver's ability to function and cope. Stay in frequent contact by telephone or e-mail. Send cards and letters of support. Try to visit and offer some respite, if that would be helpful. Ask the caregiver to inform you of situations where he or she could use assistance.

Perhaps the most important way you can support the caregiver is to avoid passing judgment on his or her decisions. Listen closely and ask questions about the situation, but don't assume you know everything that's happening. Your emotional support and encouragement are integral.

Impact on family

As you transition into a caregiving role, you may find other aspects of your life receiving much less attention. There may be little time and energy to share with your family or direct toward your spouse. Rather than feel guilty or trapped in these circumstances, look for ways to integrate the various aspects of your life. Be open and honest about your situation and accept support when it's offered. Use patience and good humor to replace tension and stress.

- Consider having regular meetings to update family members about your loved one's condition and the challenges that both of you face. Because this is a progressive disease, the others may not be aware of current circumstances and are surprised by the changes.
- Recognize that as the primary caregiver, you generally have the best understanding of the situation. Your insight may be a critical factor in many care and treatment decisions. Listen closely and respond to family questions, but at the same time, make sure your voice is heard.
- Provide family members with an opportunity to help out if they're willing to do so. Create a list of needs for your loved one and for you. Work with family members to delegate tasks, but only to an extent that they feel comfortable with.

Overcoming denial

Most family members want to be supportive but some may experience denial about the diagnosis or minimize the impact of the disease on you and your loved one. Denial is a natural reaction that people may have to buffer themselves from painful news. Family members in denial may question your judgment and discourage you from using essential resources. Try to share information with them, but recognize that you may never be able to convince them about the realities of the disease.

Sharing a doctor's written report that details your loved one's diagnosis may help. But the best way to convince people in denial is to have them spend more time with your loved one.

- A good rule of thumb is to assign a person's involvement in decision making in proportion to the amount of time that person spends in caregiving. For example, if a wife cares for her husband 90 percent of the time, she should have 90 percent of the decision-making power. If a family member isn't able to devote direct time to caregiving, he or she may offer opinions for consideration but should not play a major role in making a final decision.
- Be open about the disease with young children and teenagers. They deserve some explanation for the physical and behavioral changes they may be observing.

Some families find it helpful to meet with a social worker, psychologist, nurse or other professional with specific knowledge about the disease. These specialists can assist you in planning for the future, identifying needs and making decisions.

To locate a professional who specializes, for example, in Alzheimer's disease, ask your doctor for a referral or contact your local Alzheimer's Association or Area Agency on Aging.

Intimacy

When you care for a spouse with dementia, your sexual relationship will change. Your loved one may experience an increase or a decrease in sex drive due to effects of the disease or of its treatment. At the same time, you may experience changes in sexual desire as you take on more roles and responsibilities — your part of the relationship may feel more parental. You also may be uncertain if your loved one is capable of consenting to sex. Take it slow and use your instincts to determine whether the experience is pleasurable for both of you. If either partner becomes uncomfortable with the experience, it should not happen.

Regardless of your loved one's impairment, touch is a powerful tool that you can use to communicate affection and reassurance. Touch can be experienced in many ways, including holding hands and hugging. When used during conversation, touch can indicate that you see and hear your loved one and you care about what's being said.

12 steps for caregivers

Following statements may provide valuable support and inspiration as you assume the role of a caregiver:

1. Although I cannot control the disease process, I need to remember that I can control many aspects of how it affects my loved one and me.
2. I need to take care of myself so that I can continue doing the things that are most important.
3. I need to simplify my life so that my time and energy are available for things that are really important at this time.
4. I need to cultivate the gift of allowing others to help me because caring for my loved one is too big a job to be done by one person.
5. I need to take one day at a time rather than worry about what may or may not happen in the future.
6. I need to structure my day because a consistent schedule makes life easier for me and my loved one.
7. I need to have a sense of humor because laughter can help put things in a more positive perspective.
8. I need to remember that my loved one is not being "difficult" on purpose. Rather, the behavior and emotions are distorted by the illness.
9. I need to focus on and enjoy what my loved one can still do rather than constantly lament what is gone.
10. Increasingly, I need to depend upon other relationships for love and support.
11. I need to remind myself frequently that I am doing the best I can at this moment.
12. I need to draw upon any higher power that I believe is available to me.

ACTION GUIDE

Used with permission from "Twelve Steps for Caregivers," Farran & Keane-Hagerty, *American Journal for Alzheimer's Care & Related Disorders & Research* (Nov./Dec. 1989).

Making a care plan

It's important to put your loved one's personal, legal and financial affairs in order soon after the diagnosis of dementia is made. Developing a care plan for the years ahead affirms your loved one's wishes regarding future treatment and care, makes you aware of the social and financial resources available to you, and clarifies your legal rights and authority as a caregiver.

You may be the primary instigator of this planning effort but it's best to include your loved one in the process as much as possible. In the early stages of the disease, people with dementia often are cognizant enough to participate in these decisions. Sit down with your loved one — if he or she is still able to participate — and over the course of several sessions, attempt to learn what you can by way of simple, direct questions. The process is something that shouldn't be rushed. You may need to consult family members as well as a physician, attorney or financial planner.

The following information about your loved one may be necessary as you start to prepare a care plan:

- Social Security and Medicare numbers
- Bank account and credit card account records, including account numbers
- Will, advance directives and burial arrangements
- Insurance records for life, health, homeowner and auto policies, including policy numbers
- Retirement benefits including pensions, annuities, Social Security, IRAs or Keogh plans
- Stock and bond certificates
- Real estate deeds and mortgages
- Vehicle titles
- Consumer loans and outstanding debts
- State and federal income tax records
- Safety deposit boxes and keys
- Contact information for individuals such as lawyers, accountants, bankers and insurance agents

Preparing for future decisions

How your loved one would like to spend his or her final days and whether or not measures should be taken to extend life are extremely important issues to decide once a diagnosis has been made. Here are the means to communicate this:

Advance directive. This legal document, also known as a health care directive, allows your loved one to express his or her wishes regarding the use of certain kinds of medical care and life-sustaining procedures. The document takes effect at a time when your loved one is unconscious or too sick to communicate and participate in life-saving decisions. There are two types of advance directives to consider: Durable power of attorney and living will.

Durable power of attorney. This is a legal action that grants a person (known as a proxy) the authority to make decisions for someone else. For example, you have the authority to act for a loved one who is incapacitated by dementia. Often, power of attorney is granted for managing money and property, but there's also power of attorney for health care. The person granting power of attorney must be cognizant at the time this action is put in writing. The word *durable* means the proxy's authority continues even at the time when your loved one is no longer competent.

Living will. This document specifies the medical treatments that your loved one wants or doesn't want at the end of life. This may involve issues such as resuscitation, mechanical ventilation and nutrition and hydration assistance. In order for a living will to be legally binding, it must conform to the statute (often called natural death act) in the state in which your loved one resides.

Conservatorship. Also known as a guardianship, this proceeding grants a conservator, or guardian, the right to make decisions and care for an individual who has been determined legally incompetent. A judge generally will make the appointment. This recourse should be considered if your loved one is no longer cognizant and able to grant power of attorney.

ACTION GUIDE

Taking steps

You may want to enlist the help of an attorney to help you and your loved one prepare an advance directive, although this isn't a requirement. Your doctor or hospital staff can provide the necessary forms and resources explaining relevant state law. You also can obtain state-appropriate forms on the Internet.

Advance directive forms should come with directions. If you have questions, ask your doctor or an attorney for help. Whoever is the proxy may be required to sign an acceptance form. Generally, you need to have witnesses or a notary present.

Once the necessary forms are filled out, make sure that everyone — the proxy, spouse, adult children, doctors and lawyers — has copies or knows how to get them. At home, keep a copy accessible.

Have a backup plan

Caregivers worry about what will happen to their loved one if they're unable to provide care due to illness, injury or death. It's a good idea to be proactive and explore your options early.

- Consult family members to create a backup plan, taking into account schedules, capabilities and desire to help.
- Contact local care facilities to find out if you can complete paperwork to have on file for quick admission.
- Inquire if local care facilities will provide short-term respite care if you become ill or need surgery.
- Enlist in a program in which someone calls your house once a day to make sure you're well, or touch base with a friend at the same time every day.
- Consider using a medical alert system that will provide you with a bracelet with a call button in case you experience a medical emergency.
- Keep a house key with someone you trust who doesn't live in your home.
- Make a list of important information that an emergency caregiver would need to know.

When your loved one can no longer manage money

Because dementia causes severe impairments to memory, judgment and reason, the disease makes people vulnerable to financial abuse. Your loved one may give away or spend large sums of money. You may discover overdue notices, or bills that have been paid several times. Your loved one may not recognize if someone is taking advantage of his or her finances. To protect your loved one's assets:

- Keep a close eye on bank account balances. Is your loved one withdrawing large amounts of cash or writing a lot of checks? Alert someone at the bank and inquire whether this person can help watch for unscrupulous behavior and contact you if he or she notices suspicious activity.
- Keep watch for signs that your loved one may be purchasing large quantities of the same item or stowing cash in hiding places around the house.
- Make sure someone reliable has been appointed with durable power of attorney for financial matters. If the disease prevents your loved one from making the appointment, consider becoming a financial conservator or guardian.
- At some point, you'll need to take away your loved one's access to cash, bank accounts and financial decision-making. This should be done at the time you notice your loved one is confused about balancing checkbooks and paying bills or is exercising poor judgment in spending.
- Some caregivers feel reluctant to assume financial responsibility for a parent or another family member. Remember that you still have your cognitive functions, while your loved one may not. It's essential that you step in to help even if the disease prevents your loved one from recognizing this need.
- Most people with dementia feel more secure if they continue to have a few dollars in cash in their wallets or purses. Provide your loved one with a small amount of cash, but don't give the person more than you feel comfortable losing.
- Contact your local Area Agency on Aging, Alzheimer's Association or caregiver support group for assistance in taking over financial matters.

ACTION GUIDE

Your financial assessment

The costs associated with caregiving can run high. The Alzheimer's Association reports families spend, on average, close to $175,000 on caregiving throughout the course of the disease. Personal savings, investments and property generally are sources of income to help meet these costs. You or your loved one also may be eligible for certain financial services that will help defray expenses. It's vital for you to be aware of all these sources.

As you prepare to assume control of the financial aspects of your loved one's care, consult with a financial planner, an attorney who specializes in estates or a knowledgeable accountant regarding the payment plans for various care alternatives. Find out if you can gift money or assets to others because there are specific laws regarding this. You may also want to find out how much money the spouse may keep and how best to utilize the financial resources available to you.

Before meeting with the financial consultant, compile all of the important information about your loved one's assets. Consider potential expenses associated with caregiving, including medical visits, prescription medications, care services and supplies. Work with your consultant to create strategies for handling investments and assets and to identify financial resources.

If you plan to use home health services or another alternative living arrangement, discuss the types and amounts of payment with the agencies before enrollment. Each care option may have specific requirements regarding the type of payment they'll accept.

Financial services

Financial services that may be available to assist you include health insurance, retirement benefits, veterans benefits, tax credits and special programs through the Social Security.

Health insurance options. Government-funded insurance such as Medicare and Medicaid — known in some states as medical assistance — and private insurance are among the financial options you may use to pay for medical care and services.

Medicare. Medicare is a federal health insurance program for people age 65 and older who are receiving Social Security benefits.

The program covers some costs associated with dementia, including portions of diagnostic procedures as well as follow-up visits. Under specific circumstances — when your loved one requires skilled care for a condition that is capable of improving — Medicare will cover some costs. Medicare does not pay for elder care or respite care, prescription drugs, incontinence supplies, vitamins, or nutritional supplements.

Medicare will pay for up to 100 days of nursing home care but, again, only under special circumstances. Your loved one would have to have been an inpatient in a hospital for at least three days in the last 30 and now must require skilled care daily for the same condition for which he or she had been hospitalized. Meeting these specifications can be difficult, and most people who apply don't receive the full 100 days of coverage. Medicare will also pay for hospice services, which are available during the last months of life. For more information go to *www.medicare.gov*.

Medicaid. Medicaid is known in some states as medical assistance. The program helps pay medical costs for low-income Americans. Since Medicaid is a federal program administered by individual states, the benefits and eligibility requirements vary from state to state. If your loved one is eligible, most nursing home costs will be covered, along with many other medical care fees. It's important to plan ahead, even if you still care for your loved one at home. Check with your social services agency for more information. Also visit *www.cms.gov*.

Private insurance. Private insurance plans vary dramatically in scope and benefit. Some long-term-care insurance policies will pay part of the cost of a nursing home but may stipulate the reason for admission and the goal of care. For example, some policies only pay for assistance in a nursing home that's expected to improve your loved one's condition, such as treatment for a broken hip.

Talk to your insurance agent about the policies your loved one owns. Be aware that good health is often a prerequisite for obtaining a policy. Once a loved one receives a diagnosis of dementia, you may not be able to add any health insurance, long-term-care insurance or life insurance policies. And the earlier you enroll, generally the lower the premiums.

ACTION GUIDE

Veterans Administration. If your loved one is a veteran, check with the Department of Veterans Affairs (VA) and your local VA hospital. He or she may be eligible to stay at a VA hospital rather than a nursing home. The VA may also help pay for up to 6 months of care in a nursing home or provide respite or family support services. Your local member of Congress can help you secure benefits from the Department of Veterans Affairs if necessary. For more information, visit *www.va.gov*.

Tax credits. Certain expenses for care or medical treatment may be tax-deductible for your loved one, or for you if you claim your loved one as a dependent. For example, if you work and need to use respite care, you may be able to receive a deduction for part of that cost. Certain nursing home costs that aren't covered by Medicare or Medicaid also may be deductible.

To ensure you are receiving appropriate information about tax deductions, work with a knowledgeable accountant. Contact your local Alzheimer's Association for the latest news on tax-break legislation for caregivers. Ask the Internal Revenue Service to receive a copy of the booklet Tax Breaks for Older Americans. For more information go to *www.irs.ustreas.gov*.

Social Security programs. Two special programs administered by the Social Security Administration may be of assistance to you. Social Security disability benefits are available to former wage earners under the age of 65 who are no longer able to work due to disability. Your loved one must have worked five out of the last 10 years and needs specific documentation from a physician that confirms his or her inability to work.

Supplemental security income (SSI) provides a minimum monthly income to people who are age 65 or older, blind or disabled, and who have limited assets and income. Much as with Social Security disability benefits, a physician must document your loved one's inability to work.

For more information about Social Security disability benefits and supplemental security income, contact your local Social Security Administration office or visit its Web site at *www.ssa.gov*.

Funeral planning

Although you may not wish to think about death, many families find it easier to make burial and funeral arrangements while their loved one is still alive. This may include arrangements for an autopsy. Such planning allows you, at the time of death, to be with your family and focus on coping rather than making difficult and expensive decisions during your grief.

A traditional funeral and burial can cost thousands of dollars. For this reason, many people set aside money to cover the expense of their eventual funeral. Or they enter into contracts with funeral homes and prepay for funeral packages. Either approach will work. It's up to you and your loved one to decide on which approach you prefer to follow.

If you decide to purchase a funeral package — whether it's a cemetery plot or also includes a casket, vault and ceremony — it's a good idea to shop around. There's nothing wrong with selecting a location because it's nearby, but if you check at only one place, you may end up paying too much. Call or visit at least two funeral homes and cemeteries.

A funeral home's general services may include:
- Preparation of the body for burial
- Copies of death certificates — you may need more than a dozen to settle insurance claims, social security issues and pension benefits
- Transportation of the body to the funeral home and to the burial site
- Use of the facilities for visitation or a memorial ceremony

Some people prefer cremation instead of burial. Although cremation can be less expensive, there are still many costs and options associated with it, such as a memorial spot for the urn. Ask the facility providing the cremation services about various options and costs.

For assistance, contact a funeral director or, if you choose, a member of the clergy. Some financial programs, such as Medicaid, will allow you to spend a certain amount of money on prepaid funeral arrangements.

Being good to yourself

As a caregiver you know that your support is an expression of love and respect for someone close to you. You're providing comfort and reassurance to a spouse, parent, sibling or friend who has become dependent on you. Hopefully, you're feeling some gratification for the time and effort you put into caregiving.

Nevertheless, dementia can be as challenging for the caregiver as it is for the person with the disease. Thinking for two demands most of your time and attention. You may find your life revolving completely around the needs of your loved one. You may wonder if there's any time left for a personal life. Your loved one may eventually lose the perception that there's a problem, while you continue to witness the emotionally wrenching decline.

The demands of caregiving are both physically and psychologically exhausting. At times, you may feel frazzled and overwhelmed. You may develop symptoms that signal you're under stress, such as fatigue, headaches, muscle aches and depression. It's also not uncommon for caregivers to feel guilty, socially isolated, and frustrated at the person they're caring for.

Understanding the personal challenges you may face is as important in your caregiving role as knowing how to provide quality care for your loved one. This section is intended to help you recognize these challenges and provides strategies to overcome them.

Focus on yourself

Many caregivers become so focused on the needs of their loved ones that they don't attend to their own basic needs. For example, they don't make time to eat healthy meals, get adequate sleep, and take an occasional break from the caregiving routine.

What's the result? Caregivers often become frustrated, run down and potentially burned out. Burnout is a state of emotional and physical exhaustion and low morale that often ends with the person giving up caregiving all together.

Thinking about yourself may seem at odds with your decision to be a caregiver — all your attention is supposed to be directed at someone else, right? But it's not selfish to focus on your own needs and desires — in fact, it's a fundamental tenet of a caregiver's job.

Staying healthy is the best way to maintain the levels of emotional and physical energy that you'll need to remain a caregiver for the long term. Staying motivated increases feelings of well-being and reassurance, both for you and for your loved one.

Consider the alternative — what can you contribute to caregiving if you're sick or fatigued? What kind of care will your loved one receive if you're depressed, emotionally drained and no longer willing to participate in decisions related to care? That's why it's critical for caregivers to make self-care a priority and make a commitment to their own physical and mental health.

ACTION GUIDE

Finding a balance

To avoid being overwhelmed by the responsibilities of caregiving, it's important to find balance in your life. One of the biggest challenges you may face is balancing your caregiving duties with other responsibilities — those of your family, work and social life. Very often, caregivers become so focused on caring for loved ones that they overlook one of their most important responsibilities — taking time for themselves.

To avoid potential burnout, here are some strategies you may follow to improve your caregiving skills while also attending to your personal needs.

Acknowledge your emotions. Start by accepting the fact that, on many occasions, caregiving will seem difficult and lonely. Rather than being overcome by guilt, try to recognize feelings of anger and frustration as normal. Find healthy outlets for releasing these emotions. Share your feelings in a safe setting, for example, with an understanding friend or in a caregiver support group. Go for a power walk, punch a pillow or have a good cry. But try not to

---

Warning signs when you may need help

As you spend time caring for your loved one, you may lose sight of your own needs. You may need to adjust your routine or take a break if you exhibit any of the following:

- Easily lose patience with your loved one
- Find no joy in any aspect of life
- Get angry with your loved one
- Experience a persistent lack of sleep
- Care for your loved one 24 hours a day, seven days a week
- Feel despair, anguish or depression
- Experience changes in appetite or energy levels
- Often drink or use drugs
- Have frequent crying spells
- Think about suicide

Seek help from a professional counselor if you have any of these concerns.

direct your reactions at the person with dementia. The disease is causing the changes in your loved one's behavior — and your loved one has no control over that behavior.

Set your limits. It's probably not hard to come up with a long list of things you intend to do for your loved one — but good intentions go only so far. You'll be lucky to achieve a third of that list. In fact, caregiving has no limits, which only deepens your frustration of never seeming to get on top of your "to do" list. Try to come to terms with the fact that you simply can't do everything yourself. Keep your expectations to what you feel you can achieve safely and comfortably in a day. Be flexible and willing to accept that whatever your accomplishments are that day, they're sufficient.

Take regular breaks. A valuable guideline to follow is allowing for respite time — regular breaks from the daily grind of caregiving. If you want to care for others, you need to find ways to keep yourself recharged. It's hard to maintain that energy if you're not getting enough sleep, ignoring your own physical needs and spending every waking hour focused on dementia care. Consider setting aside time for a two-hour break at least twice a week. Spend part of that time in an activity unconnected to caregiving. Even short walks, solitary time at home or a visit to a friend's home can help to revive your spirit. Without regular breaks, you'll likely burn out, become ill or lose the ability to support and positively affect your loved one's care.

Get help when you need it. Eventually, there will be times when you need assistance from others, even if it's only to do one task or to get respite a few hours a week. An obstacle you may need to overcome is your own reluctance to ask for help. You may be worried that your loved one won't feel comfortable with other caregivers. Maybe you think that no one else can provide care as well as you can.

In fact, getting help can make caregiving less burdensome, both physically and emotionally. This assistance can provide resources and skills that you may not possess and allow you to rejuvenate your energy. Your loved one's experience may actually seem to improve. This may occur because he or she is able to socialize with more people, or it may relate to your lowered stress level.

ACTION GUIDE

Managing stress

Different kinds of stress can hit a caregiver from different directions. The sources of stress may change from day to day, increasing your level of uncertainty. Common sources of stress include:
  • Having too much to do
  • Added, unforeseen responsibilities
  • Routine frustrations of daily care, which often are beyond your control
  • Changes that inhibit your lifestyle, social life and future plans
  • Feeling inadequate to the task of caregiving
  • A sense of personal loss or grief associated with the caregiving experience
  • Disagreements with others regarding care of your loved one
  • Uncertainty about what the future holds

Warning signs of stress

Recognizing the early warning signs of stress is the foundation of good stress management. Often, caregivers don't recognize stress overload until they experience one or more of these common signs and symptoms:
  • Overwhelming feelings of anger, frustration or anxiety directed at either a loved one or the daily routine of caregiving
  • Frequent headaches, backaches or colds
  • Insomnia
  • Increased use of alcohol, over-the-counter or prescription drugs, or other substances
  • Feelings of grief, hopelessness or depression
  • Diminished sense of humor
  • Loss of interest in usual community or social activities
  • Periods of crying or other emotional outbursts
  • Loss of interest in recreational activities
  • Lack of attention to physical heath — for example, over- or undereating and avoiding exercise — and becoming run down

Take time to reflect on stressors in your day-to-day experience. The following may help you develop a stress management plan:

Identify your stressors. When you're feeling overwhelmed, jot down the particular circumstances in a notebook. Realize that stress can be caused by external factors — environment, family relations or unpredictable events — as well as by internal factors — negative attitudes, unrealistic expectations or perfectionism.

Examine your stressors. Try to identify the problems at their roots. Ask yourself, "Can I change this situation?" or "Can I improve my ability to cope with this situation?" Remember that there are some aspects of your life that you can't change — for example, having to work — and other aspects that you can change — for example, simplifying your work schedule.

Select one stressor. It's best to focus your efforts on relieving only one stressor at a time. Choose one that you feel most ready to address. When you have some success, systematically move on to the next stressor.

Set achievable goals. Consider several changes in your lifestyle that may help stop or relieve your stressor. Make the change that you're most willing to make or that seems the most practical and doable. If that doesn't work, try another of your options.

Learn to relax. Develop a strategy that can help you relax whenever you find yourself becoming stressed. Some strategies are described on pages 252-253.

For example, a caregiver may feel as though she spends all of her physical energy caring for her spouse. She always used to walk with her neighbor in the mornings, and now it seems like she never has the time. This makes her upset and a little depressed. Her goal is to make time to exercise regularly. Here are practical changes that she might make to achieve this:

- Walk while her spouse is napping or arrange for someone to care for him, if necessary, for a half-hour three times a week
- Invite her neighbor to resume the morning walks, but for shorter periods — perhaps 15 minutes
- Exercise in the house. Perhaps she might purchase a treadmill or stationary bicycle or do stretching or aerobic exercises

ACTION GUIDE

Learning to relax

When you feel anxious or stressed, the normal response is arousal — your body prepares to stand and fight the threat or to run from it. Many situations in the caregiving experience can force this response and, if they happen repeatedly, may harm your health. For example, your health may suffer if you deal with a loved one who frequently becomes stubborn and aggressive.

To ease these situations, experiment with strategies to help you relax. Relaxation eliminates tension from your body and mind. By using relaxation techniques to reduce the effects of stress, many people gain health benefits, such as the following:

- Fewer symptoms of illness, such as headaches, nausea, diarrhea and pain
- Fewer emotional outbursts
- More energy
- Improved concentration
- Better ability to cope
- More efficient performance

More than skill, relaxation takes patience and practice. Don't be discouraged if you don't feel the benefits right away. They'll come. Following are some techniques that you might use to calm your mind and body:

Relaxed breathing. Also called diaphragmatic breathing, this technique helps you breathe deeply and more efficiently, even in stressful situations.

Progressive muscle relaxation. This technique helps reduce muscle tension by having you systematically tense and then relax certain muscles.

Autogenic relaxation. It's a process in which you repeat calming words or suggestions that relax you, reducing tension.

Imagery. Imagery, or visualization, is a technique in which you form mental images of places or situations that you find relaxing.

Tai chi, yoga and meditation and self-hypnosis. These are other popular strategies that may help you relax. Talk to your doctor or a nurse about relaxation skills and how you can learn them.

Simple breathing exercise

Here's an exercise to help you learn to do deep, relaxed breathing. Practice it until it becomes natural.

- Lie down on your back on a bed or couch or sit comfortably in a chair with your feet flat on the floor.
- Rest one hand on your abdomen and one hand on your chest. This will allow you to feel the natural movements of your breathing and help you control the exercise better.
- With your mouth closed and your shoulders relaxed, inhale slowly and deeply through your nose to the count of six. Allow the air to fill your lungs, pushing the muscles in your abdomen out.
- Pause for a second and then slowly release the air through your mouth as you count to six. Make each breath a smooth, wave-like motion.
- Pause for a moment. Then repeat this exercise several times, until you feel better. If you experience lightheadedness, shorten the length or depth of your breathing.

ACTION GUIDE

Thinking positive

The endless stream of thoughts running through your head every-day is called self-talk. Often critical and negative, self-talk can discourage you to the point of despair. On the other end of the spectrum is positive self-talk, which can be a powerful tool for building self-confidence and motivation. You're using positive self-talk when you climb or bike up a steep hill, repeating all the while, "I can do it! I can do it!"

Some caregivers are unable to acknowledge — or recognize — the strain on their emotional outlook. Yet the many demands of caregiving can seem thankless. Feeling unappreciated and isolated can lower self-esteem and cause negative thinking. If so, you may

---

Depression: When to seek help

It's not unusual for caregivers occasionally to feel sad, lonely and irritable. After a short time, many people can shake these emotions and begin to feel more positive. But if the feelings persist, you may be experiencing depression. The following are common signs and symptoms of depression:

- Persistent sadness
- Irritability
- Overwhelming feelings of anxiety
- Loss of interest or pleasure in life
- Neglect of personal responsibilities or personal care
- Changes in eating habits or sleeping patterns
- Fatigue and loss of energy
- Extreme mood changes
- Feeling helpless, hopeless or worthless
- Physical symptoms — such as headaches or pain — that don't get better
- Increased alcohol or drug use
- Thoughts of death or suicide

Talk to your doctor if you have any of the above symptoms for a prolonged period of time. If you find yourself thinking about suicide or making a suicide plan, seek immediate medical help.

be setting yourself up for feelings of anxiety or depression, which sap your emotional strength and diminish your ability to care for your loved one.

If you find yourself regularly being critical of yourself or your situation as a caregiver, try one or more of these strategies:

Replace negative thoughts with positive self-talk. Throughout the day, stop for a few moments and evaluate what you're thinking. Question any thoughts that you feel are upsetting. When you find yourself being critical, replace those thoughts with positive ones. You can do it with a little practice. Convince yourself that you're an essential and positive part of your loved one's experience.

Build self-confidence and self-esteem. Focus on the things you do well. Avoid self-criticism and negative thinking by giving yourself credit for the important work you do. Make a list of your strengths as a caregiver. Make a list of things you like about yourself and another list of reasons why others like you.

Share your concerns. Talk to a family member, friend, counselor or clergy member. The support you receive can be emotional — a shoulder to lean on — or it can be practical. Positive feedback can help you avoid negative thinking.

ACTION GUIDE

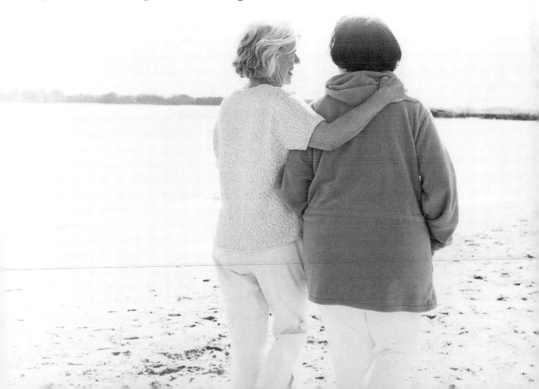

Self-care strategies

Self-care includes all the things that you do to keep yourself healthy, happy and functioning well. These actions you take can be extremely simple or complex. They range from bandaging a cut to taking blood pressure medications to knowing how to respond to a poison emergency, from routinely preparing healthy meals to regularly exercising to avoiding secondhand cigarette smoke.

Self-care is especially important for you as a caregiver because you're responsible for another person. Try to incorporate healthy self-care strategies into your daily routine. Keep regularly scheduled medical checkups and dental appointments. Monitor your use of alcohol and medications. Watch for signs of depression and manage your stress. See your doctor if you become concerned or are experiencing any signs of poor health.

From the list below, identify at least four things that you can do right now to be good to yourself. Remember, if you want to be able to care for your loved one, you need to keep yourself healthy and remain energized.

- Eat at least one healthy, balanced meal every day
- Get enough sleep
- Exercise regularly
- Take my medications as prescribed
- See my doctor for a routine physical
- Schedule regular breaks from caregiving duties
- Ask for help and accept it when it's offered
- Get support from other caregivers and share some of my experiences
- Seek supportive counseling or talk to a trusted friend when I'm feeling overwhelmed
- Maintain a sense of humor and continue to do things I enjoy, with or without my loved one

Taking care of yourself will enhance your ability to care for your loved one. Even a 10-minute walk can lift your mood, get you into a more positive environment and refocus your thoughts. Your own needs and desires are included in your job as a caregiver. Don't forget to take care of them.

Finding support

There will be times throughout the caregiving experience when you'll need assistance beyond what you alone can provide. Sources of support fall under two broad categories: informal and formal.

Informal support refers to family, friends, neighbors and faith communities. These groups often consist of people who knew your loved one before onset of the disease. They may be very reliable when you need to arrange respite care. And their home visits can be as much for your benefit as for your loved one's by keeping you socially connected. However, some caregivers report that although these informal groups are well-meaning, they sometimes drift away, leaving the caregiver without the promised help.

How can you maintain a connection with your informal support systems? Be specific as you inform them of your situation. Through a phone call, letter or personal visit, tell people about the diagnosis, the symptoms and the behaviors of your loved one. Describe your current needs for assistance and offer suggestions for the kinds of activities to do during visits.

Prepare a list of things that routinely need doing and let your "helpers" choose tasks that are right for them. Another approach is to list all of the tasks you're accountable for in a normal day. You may try assigning tasks based on the qualities and resources you

ACTION GUIDE

Using your informal support system

When someone says, "Let me know if you need something," you can give the person a list of ways he or she can help:

- Provide transportation to doctor appointments
- Call or visit once a week
- Send cards and letters that can be read aloud
- Help organize and process medical bills
- Provide a hot meal
- Shopping or errand running
- Do housecleaning, laundry or yardwork
- Inquire occasionally about how you're doing
- Be a listener or provide a shoulder to cry on

feel individual helpers can provide. Some jobs may involve physical labor while others may be directed toward paying bills or contacting local resources. Family and friends often find it rewarding to help — it's a way to show they care.

Formal support systems include any nonprofit or for-profit agency that provides assistance to individuals in caregiving settings. Formal support includes home health agencies and elder care centers. Various residential care settings may provide a place where you and your loved one can live so that you can continue to be together, or where your loved one can live in a community setting with others who have dementia.

A support group consists of caregivers in similar situations that meet to share experiences and emotions. Meetings are generally facilitated by a professional or by a trained volunteer. Attending a support group can be an opportunity for you to hear from others who have dealt with issues similar to the ones you've experienced. There may also be times when you aren't looking for new ideas or advice — you just want to be among people who understand what you're going through.

With more emphasis being placed on the early diagnosis of dementia in recent years, support groups for those with early-stage Alzheimer's are becoming more common. To join, generally your loved one must have some recognition of the diagnosis and must want to talk to others who are dealing with similar experiences.

To find support groups in your community, contact the Alzheimer's Association or your local Area Agency on Aging. Some groups may be specifically for Alzheimer's caregivers, while others may encompass broader caregiving issues.

Online support groups

You may find a variety of chat rooms and e-mail support groups on the Internet. Be cautious of information you receive from these sources. What you find may not be reliable. Use your own good judgment about the Internet and check advice with a trusted medical professional.

First person: The support group experience

Members of the Caregiver Support Group for men, ranging in age from 55 to 90, are businessmen, doctors, farmers, clergy, firemen, carpenters, teachers and veterans. They all have two things in common: Each of them has a loved one with dementia — most often, a wife — and they have decided to share their caregiving journey.

The support group meets regularly twice a month. The men find support in each other at a time when it feels like no one else understands. The group offers companionship when isolation is a common occurrence. It fosters friendships at a time when friends can be scarce. With the support of one another, the men have become more confident caregivers. They listen and learn from one another. At different times, they assume the roles of student, mentor and teacher.

Joe has been a student at times, looking to group members for answers to difficult questions. He's been a caregiver for his wife since her diagnosis of Alzheimer's disease a couple of years ago. Joe also has been a mentor and teacher. Joe showed others that caring for a person with dementia meant helping that person maintain his or her identity and sense of dignity — even if it involves something different and unfamiliar. When Joe helps his wife with her hair, makeup, and clothing, it's important for Joe to do it "just right" because his wife was always particular about that sort of thing. When Joe looked at day programs for her, he found a place that was "pretty" because his wife always liked things around her to be pretty. For Joe, caring for his wife meant respecting her for the person she had been — and the person she still is. The group learned by Joe's example.

Attending a support group didn't come easy for Joe. He's a rather quiet, reserved gentleman who feels most comfortable handling his affairs in a private way. At the beginning, Joe may have attended the support group apprehensively, as many men do. But somehow Joe found his way and has continued to attend for several years. One of the greatest lessons to learn from Joe may be that asking for help and support isn't the same thing as being needy or dependent.

Activities of daily living

The activities of daily living are routine tasks that everybody performs in order to care for themselves and to stay healthy. These activities include such things as bathing, grooming, dressing, toileting and eating. Most people expect or plan to do them everyday. When someone with dementia begins to have difficulty with these tasks — ones that were once so routine — frustration and agitation can quickly follow.

The cognitive losses associated with dementia affect fine motor skills, making it difficult to button buttons, comb hair, use a toothbrush or use eating utensils without spilling. Loss of reason and judgment that also accompany the disease make it difficult to choose appropriate clothing for the weather, to select clothing that matches, or even to put the correct shoe on the correct foot. Loss of attention and analytical thinking affects the ability to learn and to correct mistakes. Memory loss makes it likely that the day-to-day performance of these tasks will be forgotten.

Early in the course of the disease, the person with dementia may still be able to accomplish most activities of daily living with gentle reminders and occasional instruction. In time, a caregiver's help becomes absolutely essential, not just to remind the person that the tasks need to be done and how to do them but also to manually perform them.

Still, the presence of a second person for tasks that can be quite intimate may feel to a loved one like an intrusion, increasing the stress of the moment. Even when it's handled in a gentle, supportive manner, the response to a caregiver's assistance may be anger, stubbornness and unwillingness to participate, and perhaps even aggressive behavior and striking out.

As you assist your loved one with daily activities, these guidelines may make the experience less frightening and burdensome for the both of you.

Take your time. Your loved one may have trouble remembering all of the steps involved in getting dressed or brushing teeth. Trying to rush things will just add to the confusion and slow the process down. Go slowly and, if you give instructions, break tasks down into a series of simple steps.

Keep it familiar. Try to stay with the same routine your loved one has used in the past. Did your mom always bathe in the evening? Keep it that way. A familiar schedule can make the process easier for both of you. Of course, everyone has good and not-so-good days. Try to be flexible if she isn't comfortable with the task at the usual time.

Participate together. Involve your loved one in tasks as much as possible. He or she still can choose an outfit if given two choices — rather than a closetful of clothes. Your loved one may be able to use a toothbrush if you demonstrate the motion. If nothing else, have your loved one hold an object while you provide care.

Be respectful. Whether it's helping your loved one with feeding or toileting, make sure his or her dignity is being preserved as much as possible. Even if you're providing full assistance, your loved one may still feel the actions are very personal and private. Keep doors shut during dressing and bathing. Use a napkin to keep your loved one clean while feeding.

Be reassuring. If a particular task is frightening or upsetting to your loved one, respond to the emotion with a calm voice and steady manner. Reassure him or her with understanding and empathy, not reason. Try to distract your loved one by singing a favorite song, telling a story or providing a snack. But be careful with how intense your distractions are. Sometimes, they may overstimulate the person. Use your discretion.

As the disease progresses, the symptoms of dementia will likely worsen over months and years. But situations also change from day to day, and strategies that work today may not work tomorrow. Be willing to take each day as it comes and try different strategies if you need to. Perhaps you might even retry ones that had failed in the past — they may surprise you.

Have patience with your loved one and with yourself. Remember, you're forging into new territory in your relationship.

Bathing and grooming

As dementia progresses, your loved one likely will go from needing reminders to bathe, to requiring hands-on assistance, to being totally dependent on others. He or she may find the experience frightening or confusing. Here are some tips to help you:

- Try to maintain a routine. For example, make sure your loved one has a bath at the same time of day. Consider a time when your loved one has the most energy — usually in the morning.
- Prepare everything in advance. Have the bathing supplies at hand and bathwater ready.
- Make sure the room temperature is warm enough to be comfortable without clothing. Keep extra towels and a robe handy.
- Provide adequate time for each task. Avoid rushing.
- Give simple instructions or commands. In a gentle tone, tell the person what you're going to do, step by step.
- Allow him or her to participate as much as possible, even if it's simply holding an extra washcloth.
- Provide for privacy. If mirrors are distracting, cover them. A towel wrapped around the shoulders or placed on the lap also may help.
- Ensure adequate lighting, but you can dim the light slightly to create a relaxing atmosphere.
- Encourage your loved one to smell the shampoo and soap to trigger a sense of enjoyment.
- If your loved one refuses a bath, back off and try again later. Consider a sponge bath or a bed bath using no-rinse soap if the refusal is consistent.
- Place nonslip strips on the tub or shower floor. Consider installing grab bars for safety. Check with a medical supply company for a shower chair or handheld showerhead, if either may assist you.
- Hair care and shaving may be done during the bath. Trim fingernails and toenails as necessary.
- Apply lotion to any areas of dry skin. Avoid using powder except lightly under the arms. Powder tends to cake in body creases.

Dressing

Your loved one will have increasing difficulty with choosing what clothing to wear. There will be problems taking off and putting on various articles of clothing. Buttons, zippers, snaps and buckles may cause considerable frustration. To make everyone's life easier:

- Emphasize comfort over appearance. Look for items that are durable, can be easily cleaned and have easy fasteners or elastic waists. Replace challenging fasteners with Velcro. Add a keychain ring to zippers for easier maneuvering.
- Try to dress at the same time each day so that it becomes part of the daily routine.
- Buy clothing a size larger than usual if dressing is difficult.
- Avoid overwhelming your loved one with clothing selection. Provide just two choices rather than several.
- Hang coordinated outfits together, or buy clothing that will always match.
- If your loved one wants to wear the same outfit every day, launder it in the evening or buy multiples of the same item.
- Lay out clothing in the order it's put on, for example, undergarments, blouse or shirt, pants, socks and shoes.
- Avoid nylon stockings.
- If your loved one needs prompting, provide clear instructions, one step at a time. Demonstrate if necessary.
- It's common for a person with dementia to want to layer items of clothing. Generally he or she will remove extra pieces of clothing if it becomes too hot or uncomfortable.
- Be tolerant of mismatched or stained items or clothing worn inside out.
- Undershirts may be used in place of bras if extra support is not required.
- Consider the possibility that your loved one may be in pain if he or she resists moving arms or legs to put on clothing.
- If your loved one consistently refuses to change clothes, provide comfortable outfits such as sweat suits, which can be worn during the day and while sleeping.

ACTION GUIDE

Eating and nutrition

Although nutrition may seem to have little effect on dementia, it's essential for your loved one to have a balanced, healthy diet. Malnutrition and dehydration may increase confusion and stress, trigger physical problems, and reduce your loved one's ability to cope with changes brought on by the disease.

In the early stages of dementia, a person — especially one living alone — may forget to eat or how to prepare meals. As the disease progresses, the person may forget table manners and eat from others' plates or out of serving bowls. Sometimes, the person loses impulse control and tries to eat anything in sight, including items not intended as food.

In late stages of the disease, loss of appetite is common. At this time you should allow your loved one to eat for pleasure. Provide foods and liquids that are appealing and easy to ingest — there should be few dietary restrictions. During the end stages of the disease, he or she may lose the ability to chew and swallow and experience choking from food caught in the throat.

To help you meet your loved one's nutritional needs:

- Be aware that his or her appetite may decrease as the day goes on. Offer food when he or she has the most energy and make the most of favorite mealtimes.
- Serve meals in a relaxed, comfortable place. If possible, eat your meal at the same time as your loved one does.
- Make every effort to let your loved one feed himself or herself.
- Don't force your loved one to eat. Follow his or her wishes.
- If your loved one becomes full after a few bites, try serving small amounts of food more frequently, or serving foods higher in calories and proteins.
- Mix foods in a blender or food processor to make them easier to swallow.
- Use straws and cups with lids to make drinking easier.
- Use finger foods if the person struggles with utensils.
- Avoid any tasks just before mealtimes that upset or frustrate your loved one.

Failing to eat

- In early stages of dementia, provide simple reminders to have a meal. For example, phone your loved one when it's about time to eat.
- If your loved one lives alone, leave step-by-step instructions on how to prepare a simple meal.
- Stay with your loved one through an entire meal.
- Demonstrate the steps involved in eating, or give one-step, easy-to-follow commands.
- Provide adequate time for meals. Avoid rushing.
- Serve simple foods that don't require utensils.
- Leave finger foods within easy reach throughout the day.
- Serve several small meals during the day.
- Make sure the eating area has good lighting.
- Reduce background distractions such as the television.
- Display foods on attractive table settings. Offer familiar foods that have varied textures, colors and flavors.
- Use contrasting colors to help your loved one locate food. For example, use a blue placemat and white plate with dark foods. Avoid putting mashed potatoes on a white plate.
- Unless your loved one's weight is a significant problem, don't discourage eating sweets.
- When preparing nutritional shakes, blend them with fresh fruit and ice cream to improve the flavor.
- Try having the person smell lemon or peppermint oils before a meal because this may stimulate appetite.
- Consider a medical checkup to see if depression, ill-fitting dentures, a medical condition or medication may be causing the decrease in appetite.

Eating too much

- Keep food out of sight except at mealtimes.
- Dish food onto plates instead of placing serving bowls on the table.
- Cut food into bite-size pieces to avoid choking.
- Remove small nonedible items from the environment.
- Demonstrate patience if the person eats from others' plates.

ACTION GUIDE

Toileting and incontinence

As with other activities of daily living, your loved one will require assistance with toileting as the dementia progresses. The caregiver may face special challenges due to the inherently private nature of the activity and to sanitary concerns. But the same rules apply when providing help: patience, calmness and understanding.

Many people with dementia begin to experience incontinence, the inability to control their bladder or their bowels. Incontinence may occur for a variety of reasons. If this is a new behavior, consider what's caused this change. Has your loved one forgotten where the bathroom is located? Is your loved one having difficulty with unfastening clothing? Is there a medical reason for the incontinence, for example, a bladder infection, medication change or prostate difficulty? If none of these reasons appears to be causing

ACTION GUIDE

Incontinence products

A variety of incontinence products can ease your loved one's discomfort. Check on their availability at your local drug store.

- Small pads similar to those used for menstruation may be placed in underpants if your loved one is experiencing urinary incontinence only. Specially designed incontinence briefs are best if your loved one has fecal incontinence or if the small pads aren't adequately holding the urine. Depending on the incontinence pattern, some people use pads during the day and wear briefs at night. Your doctor or pharmacist can help determine which product is best for your loved one.

- Use a plastic or rubber pad under a fitted bedsheet for nighttime incontinence. Disposable Chux pads, which have highly absorbent batting and waterproof backing, can also be used to reduce frequent bed changes.

- At night, you may find it is easier to change pads or briefs while the person is lying in bed rather than seated in the bathroom. During the day, changing may be easiest when the person is seated on the toilet.

the incontinence, it may be occurring as a result of the disease process. Here are ways to help you cope:

- Follow a bathroom routine and stay with it as closely as possible. Provide frequent reminders to use the toilet. Generally, a pattern of every one to two hours works well. You may need to bring the person to the bathroom and provide hands-on assistance to help unfasten clothing.
- Place a picture of a toilet, accompanied by the word *toilet*, on the bathroom door. Avoid the word *restroom* or *bathroom*, which may be taken literally.
- Allow the door to the bathroom to stand open. Nightlights or motion sensor lights will help your loved one locate the room easily, particularly at night.
- Remove all throw rugs from the bathroom and from corridors leading to the bathroom. Some caregivers put reflective tape on the floor in the shape of arrows that point to the location of the bathroom.
- Watch for nonverbal signs that indicate your loved one needs to use the toilet. He or she may not recognize the feeling of a full bladder or lack the verbal skills to state an urgent need. You may find your loved one tugging on his or her pants, pacing or showing other signs of agitation.
- Often, there's little time between your first awareness that a loved one needs to urinate and the incontinence episode. Accidents are going to happen. Be understanding and reassuring if your loved one becomes upset.
- Avoid clothing with complicated fasteners. Elastic waistbands and Velcro fasteners usually work well. Women may fare better with knee-high stockings instead of regular pantyhose.
- Dehydration is fairly common for people with dementia. Don't decrease fluids unless the person is drinking excessive amounts of liquid — more than eight to 10 glasses in a day. Discourage drinking more than one beverage after dinner to decrease nighttime incontinence.
- A new episode of incontinence should be evaluated by a doctor. Specifically, inquire about tests to determine if your loved one has a urinary tract infection or bladder infection.

Preparing for the holidays

Celebrations and holidays can be extremely stressful and emotionally wrenching times for the family when a loved one has dementia. You may wonder how to plan for the season. If your loved one can't participate in large family gatherings, should the gatherings be held at all? Should you modify favorite traditions or try something completely new? Consider the following strategies as you prepare for celebrations:

Set realistic expectations for you and your loved one. You probably can't celebrate in the same way you did before your loved one's diagnosis — but you can still make the holiday meaningful.

- You may feel guilty if a loved one can't take part in every activity, but it's best to limit participation to a reasonable level.
- Mingle seasonal activities into your loved one's usual routine. Completely changing the routine or altering the look of the environment will likely confuse the person.
- Throughout the holiday season, expect to feel varying emotions. The holidays can be as painful as they are pleasurable. Fluctuating emotions are normal. Work through them by taking a break or by sharing them with a friend or support group.

Caregivers may feel pressure to do activities, visit people or travel when they really don't want to. Participate only in what you feel comfortable doing. Share your time with the people you love.

- It may be easier for your loved one to attend several small gatherings of short duration rather than one big party.
- If you have a large family gathering, control the amount of stimulation coming from music, television, conversation and meal preparation.
- Reserve a quiet room for your loved one to relax in. If it gets too noisy or active, tone things down.
- Don't be afraid to enjoy quiet time by yourself or to attend events without your loved one.

A key concept is to simplify. As a caregiver, you probably won't have the time or energy to do all the preparations and participate in all the activities you once did. Likewise, your loved one won't be able to handle lots of stimulation.

- A home-cooked meal at your house might still be an option if you ask people to bring potluck.
- Limit your baking, for example, by making two or three favorite kinds of goodies rather than a dozen varieties.
- To make things easier, consider a photocopied holiday letter rather than individually handwritten cards.

Prioritize which traditions are most important to you and which you can live without. You may need to modify some activities:

- People with dementia get worn out as the day progresses, so consider having your holiday meal earlier in the day.
- If attending religious services is overwhelming for your loved one, have family members alternate attending early or late services with staying at home.
- Avoid holiday shopping with your loved one during times when stores are most crowded. You might choose to pick out gifts from a catalog or online instead.

Other ways to modify holiday traditions include the following:

- Do holiday baking together. Have your loved one stir batter, roll dough into balls or simply watch as you work.
- Wrap gifts together. Have your loved one attach the bows.
- Read through the cards you receive with your loved one. Reminisce about the people who sent them.
- Take a drive around town to look at seasonal decorations.
- Sing holiday songs together or ask a family member to read favorite holiday stories or religious verses aloud. Play simple games such as guessing the names of tunes.
- Avoid setting out edible decorations or artificial fruits, which may be mistaken as snacks. You may want to forgo using blinking lights on the tree or in windows because they can increase confusion.
- Deciding whether to take a loved one away from a nursing home during the holiday is difficult. Try a small outing beforehand to see how it goes. Some people in nursing homes feel anxious when they're away from their familiar environments. Having small family groups visit for one or two hours over several days might work best. Consider joining holiday activities planned by the assisted living facility or nursing home.

ACTION GUIDE

Good communication

Communication is more than just speaking and listening — it also involves the tone of your voice, facial expressions, gestures and demeanor. Through communication, you convey facts, opinions, needs, desires, feelings and emotions.

New skills and new ways of communicating are required as the dementia progresses in your loved one. Learn to accept the changes that occur. Keep in mind that what you see and hear is a result of the disease, not of your loved one trying to be difficult or troublesome.

Early problems your loved one may experience often include "finding the right word" and thoughts that are left hanging in mid-sentence. Most often these are minor frustrations that can be over-come, and the ability to communicate generally is accomplished.

By the moderate stages of dementia, you may no longer be able to understand what your loved one is saying. Words and sentences have become jumbled. You may find it difficult to converse in a way that your loved one comprehends. These situations may lead to embarrassment, agitation and even aggression.

Being able to communicate with your loved one requires you to enter his or her world. In that world, the distinctions between past and present are often blurred — the person may be worried about situations that no longer apply, involving children, parents or going home. Trying to convince your loved one of the truth generally is fruitless and may be frightening to him or her. It's best to jump into his or her world and help make it less frightening. What you're attempting to do is join your loved one, not to bring him or her back into your reality.

When you're communicating with your loved one, focus on feelings and emotions in your conversations — providing comfort, warmth and reassurance. Don't get caught up with facts — too many names, dates, places and numbers. Employ nonverbal means to communicate — facial expressions, gestures and touch.

Basic techniques of communicating

No matter what stage of the disease process, basic techniques can help you communicate and interact with your loved one. Following are principles you may adapt and follow:

Be an active listener. Eyes and ears play big roles in good communication. The goal of active listening is to understand not just spoken words but also the underlying meaning that the person is trying to express — even if it's not expressed well.

Consider the environment. Some circumstances are good for communication and others aren't. Be sensitive to the sights and sounds around you. Speak in places that are free from distractions. Too much noise and activity hinders communication.

Set the tone. How you present yourself is critical. Are you nervous or frowning? Are you speaking clearly and simply? Is your facial expression or body language sending negative undertones? People with dementia may struggle with understanding the spoken word, but they're attuned to nonverbal signals and will respond to them in kind.

When speaking to a person with dementia:

- Talk naturally in a relaxed tone of voice and a pleasant, positive manner.
- Make sure you have your loved one's attention. Face the person before speaking and state who you are. Saying the person's name or using a gentle touch also may help.
- Speak at normal levels or a little louder if listening conditions are difficult. Politely ask if you're being heard and understood.
- Maintain eye contact and use relaxed body language. Let the person know that you care what he or she is trying to say.
- Speak clearly and directly, using familiar words, short sentences and simple concepts. Avoid complicated questions. Avoid logic and reason in lengthy responses.
- Respond to the emotion in the voice. If your loved one is clearly upset, it's enough to give a hand squeeze or hug and say, "I know you're feeling badly. I'm sorry."
- Use nonverbal cues, such as pointing or a smile or reassuring touch. Don't hesitate to repeat what you've said.

More tips for good communication

- Give instructions in simple steps, one step at a time. As each step is completed, give instructions for the next step.
- Ask simple questions, one at a time. Avoid leading questions that include the answer with it — "You're comfortable, aren't you?" The person will likely agree with anything you say.
- Allow plenty of time for a response. Two or three minutes may be needed before your loved one can even begin to answer a question. Rephrase your question if the person is unsure about what has been asked.
- Don't interrupt his or her speech. A person with dementia may require extra time to express what he or she wishes to say. Gently provide the word or phrase if the person is struggling to express a thought.
- Use a best-guess strategy if you don't understand exactly what's being said. Reassurance may count for more than absolute truth.
- Sometimes, your loved one may confabulate, that is, provide details of fictitious events that he or she will steadfastly swear are true. Consider whether it's really necessary to "correct" the truth or simply to let it slide.
- Take note of the facial expressions and hand gestures of your loved one, as they may be replacing forgotten words.
- When giving instructions, avoid statements with the words "don't," "you can't," and "that's not what I said." Instead of saying "You can't sit there," try saying "This other seat will be much more comfortable."
- Avoid criticizing, arguing or confronting. This tends to make the situation worse. A person with dementia no longer has the ability to be rational or logical, so it's unlikely that he or she will see things the way you do.
- Avoid quizzing your loved one or expecting him or her to depend on his or her memory. Instead of saying, "Do you know who this is?" try "Here is your granddaughter Susan, who has come to visit you."
- Don't "talk down to" or be condescending toward the person. Treat him or her as an adult.

First person: Communication challenges in the early stages

There are days when my husband is alert and we communicate just fine. Then there are days when it's difficult to make any connection with him.

One of the most important ways I can make him more responsive is calmness. I demonstrate this with my tone of voice, gestures and body posture. If I appear calm, he generally is calmer and our inter-actions are more positive — at least most of the time. Nothing is ever certain with this disease.

Keep in mind, calm is how I try to appear — it may not be how I feel. It's like the duck you see swimming on a pond. To an observer, the duck is floating calmly on the surface of the water but underneath the duck is paddling like mad.

Allowing my husband time to talk without interrupting him is also important. I will offer him a word if he's grasping for an idea and seems to want the help. It's sort of like a "fill in the blank" game. I want to be helpful and work with the clues he gives me but, ultimate-ly, I want him to express his own needs.

I also try to cue my husband with short, simple sentences, without seeming to speak "down" to him. My technique is to use sentences that convey one idea at a time, making it easier for him to grasp them. For example, saying, "We're going to go to the store, so please use the bathroom and get your shoes on and be ready in five minutes," will not get the desired results — at best, he'll remember to use the bathroom. It's more effective to start with, "Please go to the bathroom" — and point in the direction that it's located. When that task is complete, I give him the next step.

It can feel overwhelming sometimes to try and communicate with someone who has dementia. My support group helps me to work through the frustrations. I also have a respite volunteer who stops by each week to play cards with my husband. He loves the company. I need the time away.

Communicating in a positive atmosphere

Think of your home environment as another means of communicating with your loved one. In the same way that a person with dementia can respond in kind to your moods and emotions, so too a person with dementia relates to the home environment. If your loved one feels relaxed, comfortable and safe, your ability to communicate and interact in a positive manner increases.

- If a noisy room seems to overwhelm your loved one, shut off the television and limit background noise to quiet music — preferably without commercials.
- If your loved one becomes agitated by a group of visitors, try to limit their number at gatherings or encourage shorter visits. Advise visitors to call before they come. If you or your loved one is having a bad day, don't be afraid to reschedule the visit.
- A long hallway with lots of doors may baffle someone looking for a place to nap or use the bathroom. Provide cues to help your loved one navigate the space. Consider placing arrows made of masking tape on the floor, pointing the way to special places. Put a sign on the bathroom door with a picture of a toilet. Put a picture of your loved one as a younger person on the bedroom door — for someone who may have trouble reading, the picture indicates a personal space.
- Be accepting of the person, no matter what changes the disease brings — scolding because he or she can't find the bathroom doesn't help. Gently guide rather than force your loved one to the right location. Remind yourself that it's the disease, not the person, causing the changes.
- When outside the home, you may find it easier to avoid large, noisy settings such as amusement parks, stadiums or playgrounds with many young children. Familiar destinations may make it easier for your loved one to feel relaxed. Try not to cram too many activities into a single trip. Plan for rest periods between activities, and locate a quiet haven for your loved one to retreat to if necessary.

What's a behavior telling you?

Later in the disease process, as dementia robs your loved one of cognitive and verbal capabilities, behavior often becomes the way to express his or her feelings and needs to others. While these behaviors are meaningful, they're not intentional — your loved one isn't doing harmful or embarrassing actions "on purpose." More likely, he or she is attempting to convey a message that can no longer be explained in words.

When trying to communicate with your loved one, consider what the gestures and actions may be telling you as well as the words. For example, agitated behavior often means a basic need is not being met — pacing might mean your mother is tired, feels hungry or needs to use the bathroom.

Problem behavior also can mean there's something upsetting about the room's environment — an air draft, for example — or that someone in the room is doing something bothersome. Stubbornness and lack of cooperation can be expressions of embarrassment, frustration or anxiety — the person may fear the loss of control over his or her life. Be sensitive to these feelings. It may be more constructive to step back from what you were doing and spend time reassuring and comforting your loved one before continuing on.

A bit of detective work may help you understand what your loved one is trying to express. Try a series of simple yes-and-no questions. Try to view the situation through the eyes of the person. If your husband repeatedly is asking to go home, for example, imagine what home may symbolize to him. Home often is associated with comfort, familiarity, safety and belonging. Can you find other ways to help him feel that way? Paging through a book of old photos while wrapped in a familiar blanket and holding hands, for example, can provide some of the comforts he seeks.

ACTION GUIDE

Correcting your loved one

Sometimes, your loved one will say things that aren't true. The statement may be relatively minor, such as a wrong name or date. Other times, the mistake may feel disturbing, hurtful or embarrassing. Perhaps your husband tells a visitor that you force him to stay at home and never allow him to leave the house. Do you try to correct your husband? How do you let other people know that the statement is incorrect?

First, stand back and take a deep breath. Consider the primary goals you've set for yourself as a caregiver. How does the offending statement affect the relationship with your loved one? Is it more important to insist on the absolute truth of a situation or to help your loved one feel accepted and reassured? You may try a gentle correction, but pay close attention to your loved one's response.

For example, if your husband laughs and says, "Oh yes, that's right, we went for a walk this morning," then it's not a big deal to provide the correction. If he continues to contradict you or becomes angry, then the correction is doing more harm than good. Even if your husband isn't bothered by what you've said, you may simply be growing tired of constantly giving corrections. Ask yourself, does it really matter?

You also may wait until later to correct or clarify the misstatement with others, when you're out of your loved one's hearing range. A glance or a subtle shake of your head at the time the statement is made also may help set the record straight. Most people probably realize your loved one is confused. If the incorrect statements are being made during a doctor visit, mentally note your concerns and ask for time alone with your doctor to express them.

Support in social situations

Bustling activity, noise and large groups can disorient and intimidate a person with dementia. Reassure your loved one in social settings by staying close by and stepping in when he or she is unsure of what to do.

Preparations beforehand may help. If possible, review the names of attendees before going to a gathering. Don't hesitate to give your loved one prompts by saying, for example, "You remember our neighbor Joe from across the street."

Some caregivers carry a card that reads, for example, "The person with me has Alzheimer's disease. Thanks for your patience." This card can be shown to cashiers, waiters and others to explain your loved one's behavior without embarrassment.

Some people with dementia may feel smothered if you're overly protective. Consider beforehand how much assistance your loved one may require and try not to exceed that level. Also recognize that, no matter how much or how little you do, a person with dementia may not be satisfied with the assistance you're providing — and you may bear the brunt of that dissatisfaction.

Visiting someone with dementia

You may find the experience of visiting someone with dementia to be frightening or emotionally wrenching. Generally, the more information you have about the person before a visit, the more at ease you're likely to feel during the visit. Learn as much as you can about family and friends, personality traits, lifestyle, work history and daily routines. This information provides conversation topics.

Bring activities that can be shared — if they're at the level of the person's ability. Reminiscence is an excellent way to connect with the person. This can come from looking at a photo album, telling a familiar story, talking about a favorite pet or listening to music.

People with dementia are highly sensitive to other people's moods, expressions, body language and tone of voice. You gain their trust with warmth, reassurance and a confident smile.

ACTION GUIDE

Challenging behaviors

Some of the most perplexing changes that dementia can produce in an individual affect personality and behavior. Instead of the normally easygoing and trusting personality that had existed before the disease, your loved one may now become withdrawn and suspicious. Instead of always being gentle and polite to others, he or she may turn irritable, short-tempered and physically aggressive as the dementia progresses.

To respond to these changes, caregivers must recognize that the ways they may have interacted with their loved one in the past — before the disease — may no longer be effective or appropriate. Caregivers often need to change their communication approach and adapt their responses to challenging behaviors.

This section can help caregivers better understand the nature of these changes and offer practical suggestions for managing them. Be aware that challenging behaviors are normal and to be expected — it's part of the disease. The person who has dementia can't learn to alter these behaviors, but caregivers can learn strategies that may help reduce their occurrence.

What's a 'behavior'?
For the purposes of this section, behavior is any action that can be seen and described. Being able to see a behavior allows you to collect information about it — how often it happens, for how long it occurs and what seems to trigger it — and respond to it.

What's a 'challenging behavior'?
A behavior is considered a challenge if, for some reason, it's not suitable or acceptable to you or to others. This could mean a behavior that's dangerous to someone (such as hitting or slapping) or is damaging to something (such as breaking objects) or is unpleasant to experience (such as yelling or arguing). Several challenging behaviors may occur at the same time — such as shouting, striking out and being uncooperative.

Understanding challenging behaviors

People with dementia often lose their ability to express themselves before they lose their ability to understand. Behavior becomes a way to compensate for this loss of expression and an important means to communicate. Loved ones are seeking to have their urgent needs understood.

When your loved one exhibits a challenging behavior, your reaction may be to try and change that behavior. But remember, due to the cognitive losses, you can't reason with or teach new skills to a person with dementia. A more constructive approach is to try and decrease the frequency or intensity of the behavior.

As you consider what to do, remember that your loved one isn't acting this way on purpose. Try not to get angry or upset. Try not to label the behavior as "bad" or "a problem" — this only fosters a sense of futility in your loved one. The most likely causes of challenging behaviors are:

Physical discomfort. Behavior may be provoked by pain, fever, infection, a need to go to the bathroom, or other discomforts.

Environment. Behavior may be provoked by the surroundings: an unfamiliar place, noise, stimulating light, or uncomfortable temperature. An environment can become overstimulating or under-stimulating, either of which can lead to challenging behaviors.

Activity. Behavior may be provoked by your loved one's inability to perform tasks that are too complicated or not understood.

3-step approach to a challenging behavior

1.) **Identify the behavior.** Examine the circumstances and provide answers to the four "W" questions: What, where, when and why.

2.) **Consider many possible solutions to stopping or preventing the behavior.** Are you meeting your loved one's needs? Can you change your response to the behavior?

3.) **Try out a solution that you feel may be successful.** If that doesn't work, try another solution on your list until you find one that works.

Strategies to manage challenging behaviors

Look for a message behind the behavior. Behavior *is* a form of communication. Consider a possible cause for the behavior. Could your loved one be tired, lonely or in pain? Could the behavior be a side effect of medication or caused by the need for a bathroom?

Be proactive, not reactive. Your approach to a situation can moderate your loved one's behavior — you set the tone. Because your loved one may no longer make sense of things, he or she cues into your emotions. If you're tense or frustrated, your loved one will likely mirror that mood.

- Use a calm, matter-of-fact manner
- Repeat instructions in the same way
- Allow time for information to be absorbed
- Praise sincerely for a job well done

Have reasonable expectations. Use your knowledge of dementia to assess what your loved one is able or not able to do at different stages of the disease. Don't make demands that will challenge or frustrate your loved one.

- Don't confront or argue with the person
- Don't speak in a condescending manner
- Avoid negative phrases — "don't," "can't," "stop"

Incorporate life history into everything. The more you know about your loved one's history, the more you may understand behaviors. Sometimes, behaviors that don't seem to make sense may stem from something that happened in the past.

Problem: A woman with Alzheimer's disease always grows restless around 4 o'clock in the afternoon. As a young adult, she had loved entertaining guests and attending social gatherings.

Solution: Establishing a 4 o'clock tea time as a daily event makes the restlessness easier to handle.

Establish an appropriate level of stimulation. Regularly evaluate your loved one's response to his or her surroundings. Early in the disease process, a person will do better with some structured activity and social stimulation. Not having enough to do can lead to boredom — and dementia mixed with boredom increases the risk of challenging behaviors.

At later stages, too much stimulation becomes a riskier issue for challenging behaviors. A calmer, quieter environment with minimal activity may work better. Tactile stimulation (based on touch) often is successful — a warm blanket or a stuffed toy animal to stroke.

Offer the illusion of control. Nobody likes to feel as though someone is ordering them around all of the time — and this applies to people with dementia. If caregivers communicate in a way that makes loved ones feel they no longer can make their own decisions, anger follows. The reality of dementia is that, as reasoning and judgment diminish, caregivers must take more control and make hard decisions. However, it's possible to communicate with loved ones in ways that give them a semblance of control.

Don't take shortcuts to distract. A successful approach to challenging behaviors is known as "Join, validate, distract" (see pages 107-108). It's important to follow this three-step sequence — don't jump ahead to distract your loved one before you've taken time to join with and validate the emotions. Distraction is not effective unless the person with dementia feels as though he or she has been understood and the concern is being addressed. Once you've provided reassurance, you're more likely to redirect your loved one successfully to a new activity.

Avoid creating a behavior vacuum. It's too easy to focus on behaviors you don't want your loved one doing. Sometimes what you fail to consider is how your loved one is supposed behave — what are the alternatives? This requires you to identify and facilitate the behaviors you want your loved one engaged in. If you can find activities that are meaningful to your loved one, it's unlikely that he or she will respond with behavior that's challenging.

Operate within your loved one's reality. Remember that you, as a caregiver, must enter the world of your loved one, which may not be anchored in the present time. Trying to use logic and reason to reconnect your loved one generally doesn't work. You're seeking to join your loved one in his or her version of reality.

Reassure. Don't hold back on efforts to comfort and reassure your loved one. The emotions that are driving a challenging behavior, no matter how extreme or ill-founded, are very real to your loved one. Respond to those emotions.

ACTION GUIDE

List of challenging behaviors

Aggression. Aggressive behavior involves confrontation or belligerent action in the form of hitting, pushing and threatening. It commonly occurs as a caregiver assists with the activities of daily living, such as bathing or dressing. It's important to control this behavior before the person causes injury to himself or herself or to someone else.

Agitation. Agitation involves urgent vocal or motor actions that are disruptive and can be unsafe. Signs of agitation include shouting, complaining, cursing, fidgeting and pacing.

Anger. Anger is a strong emotional response that often shows itself in a desire to fight back at the cause of displeasure. Becoming irritable is a somewhat milder response.

Anxiety. Anxiety involves extreme fear about an impending event. The dangers can be real or imagined. Anxiety may occur for a variety of reasons. A person with dementia may worry needlessly about family, work and things left undone, even if these are no longer his or her responsibilities. Someone with anxiety may feel restless and unable to sleep.

Apathy. Apathy is the challenging behavior most commonly reported by Alzheimer's caregivers. The feeling is characterized by indifference, often in situations that would normally arouse strong feelings or reactions. Apathy may also include a lack of motivation, sitting and staring blankly, and disengagement from the world.

Clinging. Clinging often occurs from a fear of abandonment. Your loved one may rely on you completely to maneuver through the day. Even the simplest tasks may involve your participation. Your loved one may also watch your moods and expressions for clues on how to react to situations.

Delusions. Delusions are false beliefs a person may have which you can't change or modify, no matter how much reasoning you apply. Delusions often occur with Alzheimer's disease, and they may cause your loved one to become suspicious and paranoid.

Depression. Signs and symptoms of depression include anger and irritability, frequent crying spells, changes in appetite and sleep patterns, and apathy.

First person: Anger and agitation

Ted, in the early stages of Alzheimer's disease, was accompanying his wife, Maureen, to a family wedding that was a two-day drive from home. After the rehearsal dinner, sitting in the car in the hotel parking lot, Ted informed Maureen that he was ready to go home. Maureen explained that it was already late in the evening and the wedding was tomorrow afternoon. She suggested they go watch television in their hotel room. At hearing this, Ted became angry and told his wife he wasn't leaving the car. Maureen, now annoyed, told Ted that he had to come with her. Ted's agitation increased. He refused to move. "I'm sleeping in the car," he announced.

It's not surprising that after a long day in a hectic environment, Ted would be worn out and susceptible to agitation. Ted wanted to return to the comfort and familiarity of his own home. Maureen's response only made Ted more determined to stay in the car.

There are other ways to approach this situation. First, it's important for Ted to feel in control of his decisions. When Maureen said, "No, you can't," Ted became defensive. Second, Ted needs to know that his feelings are validated. Here's how Maureen could have changed her approach:

"Ted, I understand that you want to go home. It's been a long day and I'm tired, too. It's OK if you want to sleep in the car tonight. Why don't we get a blanket and pillow from the hotel room so you'll be warm and comfortable?"

Ted now is more likely to follow Maureen into the hotel room. He knows his feelings have been heard, his wife understands his request, and he feels in control. Once in the hotel room, Maureen can say, "It feels good to relax. Would you like to watch TV and order room service before you go back outside. I know I'm a little hungry." After a short time in a calm environment, Ted likely will forget his request to go home.

Frustration. People who are frustrated seem to be in a chronic state of tension or insecurity. The feelings are caused by an inability to resolve problems or fulfill needs. To reduce frustration, you can try to anticipate troublesome incidents before they occur. However, it's important to remember that frustration is a natural response to the mental and physical losses caused by dementia and you'll not be able to prevent all occurrences.

Hallucinations and misperceptions. A hallucination is seeing or hearing something that's not there, such as seeing a child in what is an empty backyard or hearing disconnected voices. The person may reach out to touch or grab whatever it is he or she sees. A misperception is seeing an object and mistaking it for something else, such as seeing a chair and thinking it's an animal or trying to pick up the flowers that are a pattern in the carpet. Caregivers should distinguish carefully between hallucinations and misperceptions in someone with dementia. Misperceptions are generally harmless. Hallucinations may be harmless but also may indicate a reaction to medication or an illness.

Hoarding and hiding things. People with Alzheimer's disease may hide objects in unusual places. This behavior occurs for a variety of reasons. Your loved one may hide items to prevent them from being stolen. The person may be concerned that he or she won't be able to find the items later and so tucks them away for safekeeping. The behavior may be reassuring if the person hoards objects he or she finds comforting. Your loved one may also collect items in the belief that he or she is still providing for the family.

Repetition. Due to memory loss, a person with dementia may not realize that he or she is repeating an action or asking the same question over and over again. Repetition may also be caused by anxiety or misunderstanding.

Restlessness and wandering. Wandering may include pacing in the home, walking aimlessly from place to place or leaving the house. It may be caused by an unsettled environment, physical discomfort, frustration or boredom. Due to confusion, your loved one may be looking for a family member or attempting to perform what was once a career-related task. You may wish to register the person in the Safe Return Program (see page 295).

First person: Clinging

Mark became a dedicated caregiver after his wife received a diagnosis of Alzheimer's disease in her early 50s. Following a year of struggle with accepting the diagnosis, Mark arranged for early retirement to be at home and care for his wife. He had a wonderfully supportive family. He participated in a support group that helped him manage his own emotional reactions and provided him with new strategies for care and activities.

His wife loved to read and would spend significant amounts of time occupied with books. As long as Mark provided for her reading activities, he was free to manage other aspects of care. However, as his wife's disease progressed, Mark noticed that she began to "puppy dog" or "shadow" him. She became anxious whenever he left the room and would follow him around the house, even as he went about his chores. Directing her to read became more difficult as she became less able to sustain her attention.

Eventually, Mark noticed himself becoming angry that he had no personal space. He could barely go to the bathroom without his wife knocking on the door and calling for him. Members of the support group also noticed Mark's frustration. They directed him to respite programs that other group members had used with their loved ones. They also encouraged him to exploit his role as a "security blanket" by identifying familiar objects that also could serve as security blankets — family photo albums, music, even stuffed animals or dolls that might give his wife a sense of security and contentment.

They reminded Mark to increase the amount of reassuring messages he provided — messages as simple as "I love you." On his own, Mark remembered that his wife enjoyed dancing. Although he himself had never liked to dance, Mark put on music and tried dancing with her one evening. He noticed that his wife seemed especially relaxed. He took it upon himself to begin a regular evening activity of dancing with his spouse. This seemed to provide her with a great deal of reassurance and relief. And, he said, "I'm finally getting a little exercise myself."

Rummaging. People with dementia may spend periods of time searching through their belongings or someone else's belongings in what may seem like a very undirected, haphazard manner. Sometimes, the person may not know what he or she is looking for. Sometimes, the thing that's being sought doesn't exist.

Inappropriate sexual activity. Sexual needs and feelings are generally a natural part of an adult's life, and they may not disappear during the disease process. Some behavior exhibited by a person with dementia may be sexual in nature, but often this behavior is misinterpreted. A lack of inhibition may cause your loved one to touch his or her genitals or undress in response to nonsexual needs, such as feeling uncomfortable or needing to use the bathroom. You may need to discreetly remove your loved one from public space.

Stubbornness and lack of cooperation. A person with Alzheimer's disease or other form of dementia may sometimes refuse to obey simple requests because the person no longer feels in control. He or she may not be willing to participate in activities such as bathing or taking medications.

Suspicion and paranoia. Doubt and a lack of trust characterize suspicion, resulting perhaps from progressively worsening memory. For example, your wife may forget where she placed her purse and automatically assumes that someone has stolen it. She may believe that whoever is in the house has taken the missing item, or she may think that someone has entered the home to steal it. Your loved one may also experience paranoia — a very strong sense of persecution — believing, for example, that people are always "out to get me."

First person: Confusion and paranoia

Katherine is in a moderate stage of Alzheimer's disease. One evening at dinner, Katherine looks at George, her husband of 46 years, and asks, "Who are you?" Although startled by the question, he replies, "I'm George, your husband." Katherine says, "Oh, that's what I thought." Later that week, Katherine is very upset when she approaches George and says, "The kids aren't home yet! They should be home by now. Something must have happened to them!" Katherine and George's children are grown up and had left home almost 20 years earlier. George, again disturbed by her confusion, takes a deep breath and replies, "The children just called to say that they're staying with friends tonight. I'm sorry I forgot to tell you. They're having a good time and said they'll see you tomorrow." "Oh," says Katherine, "That's sounds nice!"

People with Alzheimer's disease often experience delusions and paranoia. In Katherine's situation, she may not have recognized her husband because her dementia had moved her reality to an earlier time in her life. Katherine may now believe she is a young mother with children at home. When she looks across the table at her aged husband, she doesn't recognize him as the person she's married to. And it makes sense that she has become worried that the children aren't home.

George handles the situation perfectly. Although his wife's confusion makes him sad, he responds to his wife in a way that she can understand and accept. If George had tried to convince his wife that their children were grown and no longer living with them, it would only confuse Katherine more. To Katherine, the belief that she has young children is absolutely real to her — and anyone saying otherwise would only increase her agitation and produce more paranoia. When George tells Katherine that the children are safe, he accepts the realities of her disease and offers her what she needs: comfort and reassurance. A few minutes later, Katherine forgets she was worried about her children.

Living arrangements

There are many resources available to help you provide a secure, safe environment for your loved one and handle tasks in the caregiving routine. These resources can be described as a care continuum. The dictionary defines the word *continuum* as "a continuous whole," meaning a series of separate but interconnecting, overlapping parts. The care continuum includes a wide array of home health services and residential care facilities that allow you, as a primary caregiver, to create a comfortable living situation. This arrangement can be easily adapted to the changes that inevitably occur as the disease progresses.

Sometimes, having many options without a lot of information only confuses and frustrates caregivers. Too many times, though, caregivers are aware of only one option — for example, a nursing home — that they consider unsuitable for their loved one's needs. The best course of action you can take is to become aware of all of the resources available in your community and take full advantage of what they have to offer. This section briefly outlines the care continuum and provides tips that may help guide your decisions.

Keep in mind that any living arrangement you decide on will involve blending the needs and comforts of your loved one with your capabilities as a caregiver. At what stage of the disease process is your loved one in? What kinds of tasks do you require the most help with? Is it bathing and feeding your loved one, or cleaning the house and running errands? Do you still work outside the home or have other, noncaregiving responsibilities to attend to?

Regardless of your situation, remember that caregivers generally perform better with several hours of respite every week. Respite is a period of time when the responsibilities of caregiving are shifted temporarily to someone else. Respite can be arranged through informal resources such as family members, friends or neighbors, or through formal channels, such as home health services or adult day care programs. Some assisted living facilities and nursing homes also allow short-term stays to give the caregiver a rest.

ACTION GUIDE

Living at home

After being diagnosed with dementia, many people in the early stages of the disease continue to live at home, especially when a spouse or other caregiver is present. There are clear advantages to remaining at home. People with dementia often find it easier to stay in an environment that's familiar and routine. If additional assistance is required, it usually can be obtained through family members, friends and neighbors. Some communities have volunteers or professional caregivers who may be contacted as needed.

As the disease progresses, however, living at home can become increasingly difficult. People with advancing dementia, no longer able to perform many essential functions, require constant supervision. They run the risk of serious injury to themselves or causing household damage. Caregiving in these circumstances requires much more of the caregiver: greater vigilance, a total commitment of time and energy, and deep reserves of emotional and physical strength. Some caregivers are able to handle these demands.

Other caregivers, though, find that they cannot do everything alone. Eventually, they begin to think about other long-term care options. This may involve regular visits by a home health aide. Or it may mean moving a loved one into a nursing home that can provide 24-hour medical attention. Whatever the decision, a change doesn't mean the caregiver has failed in any way.

Impact on the caregiver

If you decide to change your loved one's living arrangement, one of your options may be having your loved one come to live with you or with another family member. This option deserves a careful, objective assessment before it takes place. Private time with your immediate family will diminish, and finding a safe haven away from caregiving duties may be next to impossible. Sleep deprivation is common for caregivers living with their loved one. You may become frustrated and have difficulty hiding your feelings. Make sure you have a support network. You might consider respite for short-term breaks.

ACTION GUIDE

Living alone

All people with dementia will eventually lose their ability to live alone because of safety concerns. If your loved one lives alone at the time of the diagnosis, you may be put in a position of deciding at what point to change his or her living arrangements. This can be one of the most difficult decisions for families to make throughout the entire disease process. Following are some guidelines that may help your decision:

Be timely and anticipate the change. Some caregivers wait for a crisis before looking at other housing alternatives. Your loved one's health and your own health are unpredictable — don't let the crisis make your plans for you. Find out what resources are available in your community before you have need of those services.

Get opinions from others. While considering your options, try to include the opinions and feelings of other family members, medical professionals and people involved in your loved one's day-to-day existence. Their perspectives and support will be valuable during times of transition.

Consider the health of the primary caregiver. Whether or not this is you, include the health and well-being of the primary caregiver in any decision that you make. Determine if additional in-home resources could relieve stress and meet the needs of your loved one. If the primary caregiver is the one responsible for all aspects of care, you may need to consider admitting your loved one to an assisted living facility or a nursing home in order to ease the burden on the caregiver.

Don't feel guilt. If you decide not to live with your loved one or to move your loved one out of the home, it doesn't mean you love him or her any less. You're choosing to let others help you provide care so that you can focus on other aspects of your relationship.

Key questions

When assessing whether it's safe for your loved one to live alone, ask yourself the following questions:

- Would your loved one know what to do in an emergency? Can he or she recognize a dangerous situation like fire or cold — or even a power outage? Does your loved one know how to get help or use the telephone?

- Is your loved one's independence being maintained at the expense of other physical, emotional and social needs? Can your loved one stay clean? Is the home environment picked up and hygienic? Is there some opportunity for social interaction?
- Is your loved one putting himself or herself in potentially harmful situations? Does he or she insist on pursuing activities that may need supervision, like cooking, appliance repair, sewing and woodworking? Would your loved one give freely to people at the door or on the phone asking for money?

When is the right time to change living arrangements? There's no clear answer. It's different for every family. You know the situation better than anyone else. Rely on your instincts, but don't be afraid to ask for the help of family, friends and professionals who can assist you. You'll need their support.

ACTION GUIDE

Safety concerns

These warning signs may signal that your loved one can no longer live alone:

- Persistent feelings of anxiety and fear of being alone
- Wandering away from home and becoming disoriented
- Stove burners left on in the kitchen
- Food left sitting out on the kitchen counter
- Food in the refrigerator not fresh and well covered
- Medications not taken reliably
- Strong odors or evidence of incontinence
- Not dressing appropriately for the weather when leaving home

Admitting your loved one to an assisted living facility or nursing home may become unavoidable if:

- There's need for skilled medical care, such as a hookup to an IV or oxygen, wound care or frequent injections
- Your loved one breaks a hip or becomes bedridden
- The primary caregiver is unable to provide care due to burnout, illness or death

Home health services

A variety of services are available to assist you in your home by means of home health agencies. These services may include skilled medical care, personal care such as bathing and dressing, and support services such as light housekeeping, meal preparation and errand running. The types of services will vary from one agency to the next.

Some family caregivers are reluctant to bring "strangers" into their home to help. But, from a different perspective, doing so may extend the amount of time your loved one is able to stay at home. By using in-home assistance, caregivers reduce the risk of burnout, which can lead to nursing home placement. Many caregivers also find that their loved one benefits from a relationship with an in-home worker. And caregivers benefit from the opportunity to receive a break from their responsibilities.

Because home is so familiar and predictable, it may be an ideal place to arrange for other people to provide care to your loved one. Following are types of in-home services that may be available, depending on your need:

- Homemakers may provide help with house cleaning, meal preparation, laundry, shopping and errand running, and medication reminders (although they cannot administer drugs).
- Home health aides provide hands-on assistance with bathing, grooming, toileting, dressing and eating.
- Nurses may assist with injections, giving medications, and intravenous therapies; wound care; applying ointment or lotions, assessing blood pressure; and using equipment.
- Occupational therapists may be available to assess safety in the home, recommend equipment such as grab bars and shower chairs, and create an activity schedule.
- Physical therapists may help someone to recover from a secondary condition such as a stroke or hip fracture.

Medical equipment may be available through the home health agency. You might need bed pans, commodes, walkers, wheelchairs, incontinence products, oxygen respirators and nebulizers, all of which might be helpful at some point in the disease process.

Handyman services, including minor household repairs and yard work, may be provided by certain home health agencies.

Specialized in-home

Meals on Wheels delivers hot, nutritious food directly into the home. Meals generally are provided once each day on weekdays. Some communities offer a group meal at senior or religious centers.

Companionship programs provide a friend to socialize with your loved one, keep him or her safe and provide a break for the caregiver. Companions may engage your loved one by going for a walk, reminiscing with a photo album, bringing a pet for a visit or listening to music together.

ACTION GUIDE

If you're considering a home health service

The following questions may help you evaluate whether a particular service is right for you:

- How long has the agency been in business?
- Is the agency certified by Medicare? If so, that means it meets federal requirements for health and safety.
- Is the agency licensed by the state? Most states — but not all — require agencies to be licensed and reviewed regularly. These reviews can be obtained from the state health department upon request.
- What is the professional training of the staff?
- What are the duties of the person working in your home?
- Is there a written plan that explains what services will be provided and fees charged? Documents should be given to you before service begins.
- What procedures does the agency have for emergencies? Are caregivers available round-the-clock?
- How does the agency protect personal information?
- Is the agency approved by your health maintenance organization (HMO) or supplemental insurance?

To locate home health services anywhere in the country, contact the Eldercare Locator line at (800) 677-1116 or contact your local Alzheimer's Association chapter at (800) 272-3900.

Adult day care

Adult day care, also known as elder care, are out-of-home locations that provide socialization and activities for adults in need of assistance. Some programs are specifically designed for individuals with dementia. It's an opportunity to take a little time off for yourself while also giving your loved one a chance to be with other people in a safe, structured environment. Even if you feel guilty about dropping your loved one off for a few hours during the week, remember that using this type of respite care can rejuvenate you and allow you to be a better caregiver in the long run.

Adult day care staff generally consists of a team of professionals, usually with nurses and sometimes social workers and therapists. You generally can schedule time at the center according to your needs. Most centers are open from early morning to early afternoon, five days a week. Most will provide a lunchtime meal, and some will offer transportation to and from your home. Some centers also have weekend hours or nighttime hours. Adult night service offers nighttime supervision for those in the later stages of Alzheimer's and the chance for a night of rest for the caregiver.

You may wonder if your loved one would enjoy being around a group of new people. The answer isn't always easy to gauge, but you may be pleasantly surprised at what your loved one finds enjoyable, even as the disease progresses. Following is a list of services that adult day care centers may offer. Probably one center will not be able to provide all of these services, but not all services are always needed.

- Daily activities that may include sing-alongs, games, arts and crafts projects, movies, trivia and reminiscing, and pet therapy
- Counseling support for clients and their families
- Health services, such as physical exams
- Meals and snacks
- Personal care such as hairstyling, toileting and showering
- Management of challenging behaviors such as wandering, incontinence and hallucinations
- Physical, occupational and speech therapy
- Accessibility for those with wheelchairs or special equipment

ACTION GUIDE

Safe Return program

People with dementia are at high risk of wandering and becoming lost. Due to their condition, many in this situation will be incapable of finding their way back or providing a home address should they receive assistance. The Safe Return program is a source of identification for these individuals, available nationwide through the Alzheimer's Association.

Here's how the program works: Families register with Safe Return and basic information about the person with dementia is placed in a confidential database, accessible 24 hours a day throughout the United States, Canada and Mexico. Both care receiver and caregiver receive identification bracelets or necklaces containing the person's first name, an identification number, and a 24-hour toll-free telephone number. Key chains, identification cards, pins and clothing labels are also available with this information.

The care receiver and caregiver wear or carry at least one of these items with them at all times. Should the care receiver ever become lost or missing, the caregiver can call Safe Return headquarters at the toll-free number. Safe Return will fax a photo and description of the missing individual to the local police department. As well, anyone attempting to help the lost care receiver will have a phone number to call and arrange for the individual to be returned. The identification number helps assure the identity of the lost individual.

Engraved on the caregiver jewelry are the words, "I am a caregiver for (care receiver's name)." If, for whatever reason, the caregiver becomes incapacitated, others will know to provide assistance to the person with dementia.

Since 1993, when the program was started, the Alzheimer's Association reports that over 5,000 people have been reunited with their families through the Safe Return program. The registration fee is $40, and the caregiver jewelry is $5. Your local Alzheimer's Association chapter may have scholarships available to offset costs. For more information on the Safe Return program, contact the Alzheimer's Association at (800) 272-3900 or *www.alz.org*.

ACTION GUIDE

Residential care options

One option for providing care for your loved one is a residential facility other than home. An common obstacle that many caregivers need to overcome is their own reluctance to consider this step. You may be worried that your loved one won't feel comfortable with other caregivers in a new environment. Maybe you think that no one else can provide care as well as you can.

But this arrangement can make your caregiving less burdensome, both physically and emotionally. It provides other resources and skills that you may not possess and the quality of life for your loved one may actually improve in a new situation.

Alternative housing

Alternative housing refers to several different residential options that may be suitable if your loved one doesn't require the skilled medical treatment that nursing homes typically provide, such as injections, intravenous therapy and wound care. At the same time, many people with dementia need continual supervision and assistance with activities of daily living such as bathing, dressing and eating. They also may benefit from opportunities to participate in social activities. Here are alternative housing options that may exist in your community:

Adult foster care. This program licenses private homes to care for up to five adults in need of 24-hour assistance. The homes are usually licensed by a county social worker, who provides ongoing visits. Homeowners may have received specialized training and may be screened with background and reference checks. People using this service usually reside at the home full time, but some foster care homes also provide short-term respite stays during daytime hours or for overnights and weekends.

Assisted living. Some people in the early stages of dementia may be well suited for assisted living. These individuals have a moderate degree of functional impairment but are still capable of tasks such as feeding themselves and getting dressed. Assisted living can provide these individuals with a degree of independence within a safe, structured environment.

Assisted living facilities, also known as board and care facilities or group homes, are typically apartment complexes that feature private or shared bedrooms and shared kitchen, dining and living quarters. Direct assistance from the staff is available 24 hours a day, when necessary. The staff members may help with personal care, provide housekeeping services, distribute medications and organize social activities and programs. Residents can participate in meal preparation, laundry and other tasks according to their desires and capabilities. There may be short-term respite stays at these centers depending on the availability of space.

Nursing homes
People with dementia who need assistance with most or all activities of daily living and require medical care may be best served at nursing homes, which are sometimes referred to as skilled care facilities. Staff at these facilities plan and monitor all meals to ensure that the care recipients are eating well, and they offer structured activity programs.

Nursing homes may be a helpful option if your loved one is in the middle to late stages of dementia or if he or she is in an early stage of the disease but needs skilled medical care or requires significant physical assistance with walking or getting out of bed.

Some nursing homes have special Alzheimer's units, also known as dementia special care units. Ideally, Alzheimer's units should provide a quiet, homelike environment, consistent activity programming and a staff trained in dementia care. Many units do not modify care to meet the special needs of people with dementia, however, and families may be served just as well by using a nursing home without such a unit.

Continuing care retirement communities
These facilities, sometimes called life care centers, offer a range of services across the care continuum so that as the needs of your loved one change, he or she may receive more advanced levels of care within the same complex. These communities include those who can live relatively independently with others who need skilled nursing care.

Finding a new living arrangement

A variety of options are available in the care continuum. Some of these options will fit your current situation better than others, depending on your concerns and needs. Consider the following issues when choosing which option is right for you:

- What options are available in your community? Your choices, especially in rural areas, may be limited by proximity. Decide how far you're willing to travel to a location. Friends and relatives, your physician, social workers, other medical staff and members of local religious organizations may be able to refer you to specific facilities.
- Consider how you'll pay for the care. It may help to consult a financial planner or a social worker for general guidance. Compare what payment options are accepted by particular types of facilities. Remember to ask if additional fees are charged for specific services.
- Consider which of your loved one's needs are of greatest concern. Do they involve the activities of daily living, companionship or medical care? Match your loved one's prioritized needs to the services available at a care facility.
- What steps are involved in the admissions process? Ask for specific admission and discharge criteria. Is there a waiting list? How long is the wait?
- Arrange tours of more than one facility. Try to visit each site more than once and at different times of day. As you tour, observe the following:
  - Does the facility appear to be properly staffed? Do staff members seem overly rushed? Is there adequate backup support in case an employee cannot come to work? How are emergency situations handled?
  - What is the facility's philosophy of dementia care? How do staff members handle challenging behaviors? Is the facility secure in case your loved one wanders?
  - How does the staff interact with residents? Do staff members smile and call residents by name? Do they interact with residents during meals?

- Are activities offered throughout the day? Ask to see a schedule. If an activity on the list is not occurring, ask why not. See if you can sit in on a program or activity during one of your visits.

- Examine the environment. Is it clean and well cared for? Does background noise from sources such as televisions, radios, intercoms and alarms appear under control?

Call ahead to arrange for a meeting with a staff member and have him or her show you around. Ask questions to find out how the center operates. Bring a family member or friend so he or she can help you evaluate. Look for a place that comfortably fits your specific needs and family situation.

Decide on your top choice or choices. Once you've made a decision, carefully review the terms of the contract and any financial arrangements before signing. It may be useful to have a lawyer review these documents with you.

Find out about preparing an application ahead of time. Prior contact with the admissions staff can help ease the placement process in case of an emergency. Ask about putting your loved one on a waiting list. Some facilities may require a down payment when you do this, but many others won't ask for a deposit at this time. Under no circumstances are you obligated to take an opening when it becomes available, even if you're on the waiting list.

Where do I find these resources?

To locate care centers anywhere in the country, contact the Eldercare Locator line at (800) 677-1116 or contact your local Alzheimer's Association chapter at the toll-free number (800) 272-3900. You can also check your local yellow pages. Look under Aging Services or Senior Citizen Services.

Evaluating the quality of service

As you try to gauge the quality of care that a professional care-giving service provides, try to strike a balance between serving as your loved one's advocate and not overwhelming the staff with minor concerns. Keep in mind you may be limited as to how much control you have over certain issues. Be willing to let go of those issues that have a minimal effect on your loved one's experience.

At the same time, it's important for you to be included in decisions that ensure that your loved one's needs are met. The best way to make this happen is to keep the lines of communication open. Offer your input as a team member, approach staff members in a gentle, assertive manner and be prepared to listen to the reasons behind a particular approach.

Before addressing a concern with a care provider, ask yourself:
- Who does this issue concern the most?
- Is my loved one at risk of physical harm?
- How much will my loved one's quality of life improve if this issue is addressed?

For example, if your father and his nursing home roommate often wear each other's clothes, who is this practice really bothering? On the other hand, if your father becomes aggressive during bath time when in the care of a particular staff member, raising this concern can help defuse the situation.

When a change is necessary

Your loved one's safety and well-being are of primary importance. If you're seriously concerned about either, you may need to find a new environment or new facility. If you have grave concerns about a specific care provider, seek help immediately. Report signs of physical, emotional or financial abuse to the proper authorities.

Each state has an advocacy organization to investigate concerns about care providers. To contact your state's ombudsman — a public official appointed to investigate your complaints — look in the phone book or check with your Area Agency on Aging or local Alzheimer's Association. Or you may contact a social worker in adult protective services at your local social services department.

Visiting your loved one

Bear in mind that during a visit to a care facility, you're not expected to continue providing care for your loved one and no longer are required to protect the staff from your loved one's challenging behaviors. You're now part of a team of caregivers. Allow the staff to be in charge. Focus on enjoying the visits and providing love, comfort and reassurance when you visit.

- Work with the staff to determine when and how often to visit your loved one. Use this arrangement to recharge your energy and enthusiasm and to resume some neglected aspects of your life outside of caregiving.
- When you visit, expect that there may be changes in your loved one. It's naturally going to be a challenge getting used to a new environment. With time, your loved one will almost always adjust.
- Try to plan visits for times of day when your loved one is alert, active and feeling at his or her best. You might bring along something familiar to show or do, such as looking at photographs or playing music. Use these items and activities, or skip them as the need arises.
- Your loved one often cannot remember how frequently you visit or for how long. Expect to hear "Where have you been?" or "Why don't you ever visit me?" no matter how long it has been between visits.
- When it's time to leave, family members may know the best way to say good-bye. A simple "Good-bye, Mom. I have some errands to do. I'll come back soon" is usually best.
- Giving a personal item such as a scarf or cap to "keep for me until I come back" may be reassuring to your loved one.

Moving day

Once you've decided on a new living arrangement, you can begin the process of adjustment. Remember that when you use other resources, you are indeed letting go of some control over your loved one's care. Although the care from others will be different from yours, you still have a tremendous influence. Here are tips for handling the move to a new facility:

- Share with your loved one beforehand as much or as little information about the move as you deem appropriate. Experts vary on their advice to families about what to say. You should do what you feel is best. There's no one correct way to handle the process.
- You may consider breaking the news on the day of the move. Avoid providing too much explanation. Keep the statement simple: "Mom, today you're moving to a new home." Lengthy explanations often lead to frustration and argument. You're not likely to convince your loved one of the need to change his or her living situation.
- Try to project a positive attitude. Explain the move in terms the person will understand. Use statements such as, "We want you to be safe, and I'm sure you want that too," or "The home is going to help you make new friends." Help your loved one feel secure. You might introduce an in-home caregiver as a nurse or just a new friend. You might describe going to an elder care center as going to work or staying with friends.
- Acknowledge your loved one's feelings of anger, grief and loss. You may find it helpful to apologize. Thank your loved one for understanding why the move is so important.
- Try to stay calm and reassuring. Sometimes, families discover the process is harder for them than it is for the person with dementia. Your loved one may be watching you closely for signs that the situation is safe. If you're tense, the person may sense this and also become anxious.
- Try to fill out all admissions paperwork in advance so that you can focus your attention on the physical move and on reassuring your loved one.

- Ask the facility staff for advice on moving day. You may be an expert on your loved one, but staff members have probably helped many families through this difficult process. Work together to create a plan.
- Help the staff get to know your loved one by providing information about his or her personal history and current care needs. A written list is more likely to be passed along to all staff, as opposed to telling one staff member. Bring a photo album or scrapbook that describes important events, friends, trips and hobbies. You may want to leave a video or audio recording of your voice for the staff to play, giving reassuring messages to your loved one.
- Be aware that Monday through Thursday tend to be the best days for moving. Care facilities are more likely to be fully staffed on these days. Fridays may be hectic and too close to the weekend, when there are more visitors.
- If possible, bring your loved one to the new facility before lunch or dinner. The meal provides a distraction and good excuse for leaving.
- Think about decorating the new living quarters before your loved one moves in. Arrange familiar items, such as photographs and knickknacks, in the room to provide a sense of identity, security and comfort.
- Decide ahead of time how long you'll stay at the new facility. Hovering over your loved one may provide a sense of security but doesn't allow for him or her to become acclimated to the environment. Your loved one and the staff need time to become familiar with each other.
- When it's time to leave, proceed according to a plan you've made with the new caregiver. You may excuse yourself to run errands or simply say, "I'll be back soon." To avoid calling attention to your absence, you may also decide to slip out without saying goodbye.
- Be gentle with yourself. This is often the most difficult thing you'll ever do with a family member. Take some time to do what you need to feel better.

ACTION GUIDE

First person: Preparing for the inevitable

Our mother is in the early stages of Alzheimer's disease. She lives alone in the home that she and my father shared for over 40 years. Our father died last year. My sisters and I are worried about mother living alone, but the thought of moving her is very painful. How do we prepare her for this possibility?

Moving from one home to another can trigger anxiety for almost anyone, especially when it's a move from a home you've lived in for many years. For individuals with Alzheimer's disease, relocating to an unfamiliar environment can be extremely stressful, even though doing so is often in their best interests.

In making decisions about when and where to move a loved one, there are no right or wrong answers. Friends and neighbors will have opinions, but the decision to move a loved one to a long-term care facility rests with the family. And the best decision is the one made by informed family members.

Plan ahead now for the day you decide to move your mom. Explore all of your housing options, and talk to your mom — while she can still make choices — about what she wants. The best approach may not be to directly ask your mom if she would like to move because the answer will inevitably be "no." Instead, bring up the topic in a more casual way. For instance, if your mom says she isn't eating because she doesn't feel like cooking for just herself, you may say, "Wouldn't it be helpful to have someone cook your meals?" This might begin to ease her into the benefits of an alternative living arrangement.

As moving day draws near, don't dwell on it too much. For example, don't remind your mom that she's "moving in a week." On the actual day, move your mom during the best time of her day — whether that's in the morning or the afternoon. This can make the transition go more smoothly. Allow for time during the day to reminisce with your loved one, looking at photo albums or memory boxes. This activity is helpful in relieving anxiety not only for your mom but also for you.

Support groups

Caregivers and family members often appreciate the opportunity to talk about their caregiving experiences and how the disease has impacted their lives. One place this can happen is in a support group. Support groups provide a safe forum for individuals to share emotions, changes and concerns with others who are in similar situations. Support groups can be a place to vent frustrations, problem-solve challenging behaviors or even share a laugh to lighten the burden of the disease.

Support groups may be offered in a variety of locations, such as medical clinics, nursing homes, churches, community centers and senior centers. The facilitator, who may be a professional or a trained volunteer, typically runs the support group. Meetings may be weekly, biweekly or monthly, generally for about an hour. Support groups may exist in your community for family caregivers and for people in the early stages of dementia. Typically you don't have to live with the family member who has dementia in order to participate in a support group. For more information on support groups in your area, contact the Alzheimer's Association at (800) 272-9300 or *www.alz.org*.

If you're looking to share experiences but aren't comfortable in a group setting, try talking with a trusted friend, family member, clergy or trained professional. The Alzheimer's Association can refer you to family counselors who can discuss your situation with you. You may also ask to speak with a social worker or nurse at your local clinic. Even regularly going out for lunch or coffee with a friend can help reduce the stress of caregiving.

ACTION GUIDE

Hospice

Hospice care is designed for people in the final phase of a terminal illness — many may have no more than six months to live. It's a special kind of care that focuses on comfort rather than treatment and on quality of life rather than length of life. The emphasis is no longer on curing disease. Rather, it addresses two fears that a dying person may have — the fear of pain and the fear of being alone.

In order to use hospice services, you must decide to stop any life-prolonging treatments for your loved one and focus only on comfort measures. For example, you may choose to no longer employ ventilators, cardiopulmonary resuscitation (CPR), antibiotics and artificial nutrition and hydration (tube feeding and intravenous hydration). This doesn't mean you're providing assisted suicide. Rather, it's a planned decision not to aggressively treat medical illness. You can still provide pain medication and oxygen to help your loved one stay comfortable. Advance directives, including living wills and durable power of attorney for health care, can help you make these important decisions according to your loved one's wishes.

Many hospice programs are run by nonprofit, independent organizations. Some are affiliated with hospitals, nursing homes or home health care agencies. Hospice care can take place in the home or in a specially designated hospice facility under the direction of a medically trained staff. Support of the entire family — not just the person who is ill — is a core element of hospice care.

Predicting the remaining length of life can be difficult for someone with dementia. Even those people with severe Alzheimer's disease may have a prognosis of up to two years. Their survival often depends on the existence of coexisting diseases and on the comprehensiveness of care. To qualify for hospice care, a physician must certify that the person is in the end stage of the disease.

Most hospice programs offer the following types of service:

Giving comfort. In many cases, the individual remains in his or her home or in homelike surroundings instead of a hospital. Care is designed to relieve or decrease pain, control other symptoms and provide as much quality time as possible with family and friends.

This is a cooperative effort by the primary caregiver, family, friends and a team of professionals and volunteers working together to meet your loved one's needs. This team supplies all necessary medications and equipment

Providing support. Individuals in the last stages of life often prefer receiving basic care from family and friends. A nurse may lead the team and coordinate the day-to-day care. A doctor is also part of the team. Chaplains and social workers are available to counsel the family and make sure emotional, spiritual and social needs are being met. Trained volunteers perform a wide variety of tasks as needed, such as providing companionship, doing light housekeeping, preparing meals and running errands.

Improving quality of life. Caring for someone who is dying is emotionally and physically demanding. But primary caregivers and family members can take comfort knowing that hospice is an act of love that can improve the quality of life for everyone involved.

ACTION GUIDE

Travel and safety

Safety becomes a greater concern as your loved one becomes increasingly dependent on others for care. The impairment of memory, judgment, reason, attention and other cognitive functions due to dementia, coupled with the impairment of mobility, balance, vision and hearing that sometimes accompanies aging, puts your loved one at high risk of injury.

It's also true that every person moves through the disease process in his or her own way. Safety concerns vary widely from individual to individual, influenced by that unique combination of genetic inheritance, medical history and lifestyle patterns that each person carries. As a caregiver, you must adapt to the changes that will occur, based on what's safest for, and in the best interests of, your loved one.

While there's no precise template to follow that can ensure a "safe" environment for your loved one, these guidelines should apply to most situations:

Anticipate problems. Don't wait for accidents to happen before taking steps to remedy problems. If you're aware of the potential but take no action, you'll be in a perpetual state of high alert.

Modify the environment, not the behavior. Caregivers often face the choice of changing the potentially harmful behavior of a loved one or modifying the environment in which this behavior takes place. Generally, changing the environment is a safer and more productive remedy. For example, if a long flight of stairs is a growing concern, you might consider converting a downstairs room into a bedroom so that your loved one doesn't need to go up and down the stairs at all.

Keep it simple. Devices and supports should be easy to use and access — not complex or requiring new learning. It's better if these relate in some way to the person's past skills and knowledge.

Do routine checks. Schedule regular times — perhaps three or four times a year — when you do a room-by-room check for potential safety concerns.

Driving

Do you remember how great it felt to drive a car all by yourself for the first time? Driving provides a deeply felt sense of independence and self-sufficiency — and rarely will people with dementia voluntarily choose to surrender the car keys. But driving and dementia make a risky combination.

People with dementia often can't recognize when they should stop driving. They often feel it's the last thing they can do by themselves, and they want to hang on to that opportunity. The final decision generally falls to caregivers, and it's among the most difficult decisions they have to make.

Some caregivers allow their loved one to drive only in familiar neighborhoods or only when the caregiver rides along. This doesn't address how your loved one will respond if an unexpected detour arises or a child darts into the road. Other caregivers employ a wait-and-see method, thinking, "He hasn't had any trouble till now, so we're keeping our fingers crossed." If this is your plan, ask yourself what sign you're waiting for. A fender bender may, indeed, be the time for you to intervene, but a catastrophic accident could happen before that minor one does.

Driving is a privilege, not a right. Dementia impairs judgment, planning, visuospatial skills and reaction time, all of which are

ACTION GUIDE

When is it time to stop driving?

Observe your loved one's driving habits for signs of potential trouble and changes from previous behavior. Intervene quickly if you notice any of the following:

- Failing to yield or observe traffic signals
- Getting lost in familiar locations
- Problems with changing lanes or making turns
- Driving at inappropriate speeds
- Confusing the brake pedal and the gas pedal
- Being confused about directions or detours
- Hitting the curb while driving
- Making poor or slow decisions

essential to maneuver a ton of steel down the road. Families who wait too long risk injury and death not only to themselves and their loved ones but also to others.

Most specialists feel it's important to help the person with dementia stop driving as soon as possible. A rule of thumb is to ask yourself whether you feel safe riding in a car that your loved one is driving. If the answer is no, then you know it's time to take away that driving privilege.

Making the decision

When you decide it's time to stop, stay committed to that decision. It's not your fault that your loved one should no longer be driving — blame the disease. You're ensuring your loved one's safety. Here are tips to ease the transition for your loved one:

- Elicit the support of family, friends and neighbors.
- When you inform your loved one of your decision to have him or her stop driving, remember that dementia affects the ability to reason. Don't spend too much time trying to convince the person why he or she can no longer drive — you're unlikely to succeed.
- A simple statement of fact may work best, but family, friends and professionals should offer similar explanations to yours: "The doctor says you can no longer drive," or "It's not safe for you to drive because of your memory problems."
- You may decide not to tell your loved one about the decision. Some families remove the car without discussion or with an explanation such as "Your car is at the mechanic's shop."
- Your doctor may be willing to prescribe "no driving" in an official letter.
- You or your doctor may request that your loved one take a driver's test. The test results can bolster your case. Some states require doctors to report diagnoses of dementia to state transportation officials.
- Allow your loved one time to grieve and adjust to the loss of driving privileges. It may provoke frustration and anger. Try to remember that, although these feelings are directed at you, they actually relate to the disease.

Sticking with the decision

Even after you've made the decision to take the keys away, you may still need to come up with clever ways to prevent your loved one from driving:

- When your loved one asks to drive, avoid giving a straightforward no. Tell the person that you would like to drive, or you're taking a new route, or the doctor doesn't recommend driving because of a heart condition or other illness.
- Out of sight means out of mind. Park the car where your loved one can't see it. Hide the keys, and if the person insists on carrying a set of keys, provide substitutes that don't work.
- If your loved one has used a particular mechanic in the past, be sure to alert that person in case your loved one asks for help in getting the car started.
- Ask for assistance from a mechanic to disable the car. Older-model cars may be disabled easily by removing the distributor cap. Of course you can always disconnect the battery. A mechanic may be able to install a kill switch that must be deactivated in order to start the car.
- Your loved one may continue to enjoy car rides. If a familiar vehicle prompts him or her to want to drive, you may need to sell the car and replace it with a different model. Your loved one may be less likely to drive if the car is unfamiliar.
- Always offer to do the driving when your loved one needs transportation. Find other ways to make the person feel active and useful.
- Look for alternative means of transportation, such as senior buses and taxis. Arrange for friends and other family members to give rides. Check with your local Area Agency on Aging or an Alzheimer's Association chapter to learn about transportation options.
- Keep in mind that as the dementia progresses, your loved one will likely feel less need to leave his or her safe, familiar home environment. Eventually it will be more common for you to run errands for your loved one rather than providing transportation to the store.

ACTION GUIDE

Traveling

Traveling or attending events outside the familiar home environment grows increasingly difficult as dementia progresses. If you decide to travel with your loved one, here are some suggestions for making those times easier:

- If you're uncertain how your loved one will react to a long stay away from home, do a "trial run" of daylong or overnight trips beforehand.
- Simplify your vacation plans. Avoid cramming too many activities into a single day and try to keep changes throughout the day to a minimum. Plan for rest periods between activities and a quiet haven for your loved one to retreat to if necessary.
- Alert travel or hospitality staff ahead of time that your loved one has dementia. Special arrangements can be made to board planes early or to use wheelchairs to alleviate fatigue in places that involve a lot of walking.
- Your loved one may become confused about when the trip will take place and what preparations are required. You may find it easier not to talk about the trip until just before leaving. Provide reassurance: "Tomorrow we're going to visit our daughter Susan in Wisconsin. Don't worry. We've packed everything we need and I'll be with you the whole time."
- Before leaving home, consider registering in the Safe Return program (see page 295). Contact the Alzheimer's Association for more information.
- You may find it helpful to alert people you meet of your loved one's condition in a discreet manner. Bring a small card with you that states, "The person with me has dementia. Thank you for your patience." Show the card to restaurant staff, flight attendants, store clerks, cashiers and others who should be aware of your situation.
- Consider bringing another person to assist you. This may be particularly helpful at locations with public restrooms, if you and your loved one aren't of the same sex.
- Create a backup plan in case your loved one needs to return home quickly.

ACTION GUIDE

- Give your loved one a small amount of money to put in a wallet or purse, but no more money than you would be comfortable losing if he or she misplaced it.
- Bring a list of medications, insurance information and emergency contacts. Compile a list of medical facilities for each destination — available from the Alzheimer's Association.
- Provide family members with your travel itinerary and contact information.
- Bring snacks and simple, fun activities like magazines with bright colorful pictures, audiotapes or CDs, or a deck of cards.
- Allow your loved one to wear comfortable shoes and familiar clothes when traveling. Stiff, unfamiliar apparel may just add to any apprehension that your loved one is feeling.
- On airplanes, buses or trains, take the aisle seat and have your loved one sit away from the aisle to control wandering. A window seat may help keep your loved one engaged.
- Try to keep meals and meal times similar to those at home. If crowded restaurants confuse your loved one, consider taking advantage of room service.
- Bring a waterproof sheet and extra pads if your loved one experiences incontinence.
- Caregivers often find trips with their loved ones to be extremely stressful and exhausting. The person with dementia experiences anxiety and confusion away from home, then quickly forgets about the trip afterward. Using respite care that allows your loved one to stay home while you travel may be easier for both of you.

ACTION GUIDE

Making the home environment safe

There are many ways to modify your home environment that can help your loved one stay safe, feel comfortable and be able to move easily from room to room. Following is a list of general precautions you might take to keep you and your loved one safe:

- Keep a list of emergency numbers by all telephones, including family contacts, your doctor's office and the fire department.
- Use a telephone answering machine when you're unavailable to answer the phone — and turn down the phone ringer when the machine is on. You don't want your loved one subjected to possible exploitation by solicitors.
- Make sure you have a fire extinguisher and an updated first aid kit in your home.
- Install smoke alarms throughout the house.
- Install locks on all outside doors and windows.
- Keep a spare key hidden outside your home in case your loved one accidentally locks you out.
- Post a "No solicitation" sign on your outside door.

Wandering

Individuals with Alzheimer's disease are at increased risk of wandering away from home and getting lost. The wandering may be a result of hunger, fatigue or boredom. Here are ways to reduce the risk of wandering:

- Install a slide bolt at the top of doors to the outside or to stairwells, or use a deadbolt that requires a key.
- Install alarms that alert you when a door is being opened. These can be purchased for a reasonable cost.
- Some caregivers disguise doors to the outside by covering them with curtains, wallpaper or paint, or by posting a "Stop" or "Do not enter" sign.
- Take a daily walk with your loved one, or allow him or her to wander in safe areas with supervision.
- Alert neighbors of your loved one's condition so they can notify you if your loved is outside alone.

ACTION GUIDE

Securing living spaces

- Keep living spaces picked up. Clutter creates potential problems and disguises many others.
- Make sure there's adequate lighting throughout the house, particularly in areas with little natural light, such as hallways and stairwells.
- Place childproof locks on cupboards and drawers to prevent access to sharp utensils, matches, small appliances and household cleaning products.
- Install plugs, covers and plates on electrical outlets that aren't being used.

Preventing falls

A person with dementia may be at higher risk of falls due to tripping, losing his or her balance, slipping on a wet or uneven surface or misjudging the height of a step. You may not be able to prevent falls completely but the following steps may reduce the risk of a fall:

- Provide well fitting, low-heeled shoes with nonslip soles.
- Keep walkways and stairways free of clutter.
- Make sure there's at least one handrail in all stairways. If possible, steps should be carpeted or have safety grips.
- Place nightlights in hallways, bathrooms and bedrooms.
- Get rid of throw rugs or secure the edges with carpet tape.
- Move electrical cords under furniture or tape them to walls. Avoid the use of extension cords, if possible.
- Arrange furniture so that walkways aren't obstructed. Avoid moving the furniture once it's in place, as this may disorient your loved one.
- If your loved one habitually falls out of bed, move the bed against a wall or put the mattress on the floor.
- Immediately clean up any spills on the floor.
- Put nonskid decals on the bathtub floor.
- Install grab bars in the shower and use a specialized shower chair.

- Keep medications — both prescription and over-the-counter products — locked away or at least out of sight, especially if your loved one is prone to taking medications more frequently than prescribed.
- Store all household-cleaning products and poisons in secure locations, preferably outside general living spaces.
- Remove poisonous plants from the home. A list of poisonous plants can be obtained from nurseries or poison control centers. Similarly, remove artificial fruits and vegetables and other food-shaped items that can be mistaken as edible.
- Be careful with electric blankets and heating pads, which are capable of causing burns if the controls are tampered with. Avoid the use of portable space heaters.
- Never leave your loved one alone with an open fire in the fireplace. Keep matches and cigarette lighters out of sight.
- Use curtains or decals on sliding glass doors and large picture windows to indicate the presence of the glass.

In the kitchen and bathroom

- Install single faucets that mix hot and cold water in all sinks and the tub. Adjust the thermostat on your water heater to 120 degrees to avoid burns. If you have double faucets, consider color-coding them red and blue to help prevent confusion.
- Install drain traps in sinks to catch materials or valuable items that may otherwise clog the plumbing.
- Regularly clean the refrigerator, removing out-of-date or spoiled food that your loved one might eat.
- Limit stove use if necessary. When the stove is not in use, throw the circuit breaker or unplug the stove. You also can remove the stove knobs or cover them with bubble lenses.
- Use small appliances with automatic shut-off devices.
- Consider removing metal bowls from the kitchen. They could start a fire if placed in the microwave.
- Store all electrical bathroom appliances outside the room and, if possible, use them outside the bathroom as well.
- Remove the lock from the bathroom door to prevent your loved one from being locked in.

First person: Food safety

My mother has mild Alzheimer's disease. The other day she drank half a glass of sour milk, which could have made her sick. The milk had curdled and it stank, yet she drank it anyway. Couldn't she see or smell that it was sour?

Individuals with Alzheimer's disease may experience changes in their vision and sense of smell and taste, as well as their hearing and sense of hot and cold. From time to time, they should be evaluated to determine if glasses, hearing aids, or dentures are needed or should be adjusted.

However, it's important to realize that Alzheimer's disease can cause changes in a person's ability to interpret what they see, hear, taste, feel or smell. In the case of your mom, there may be nothing wrong with her eyes or her ability to smell and taste. But due to her Alzheimer's disease, she may have lost her ability to recognize that curdled or lumpy milk is spoiled. Or she may no longer be able to interpret that a sour smell or taste makes it unsafe to drink. In addition, people with Alzheimer's disease can lose some of their taste sensitivity.

You'll want to keep the refrigerator clear of spoiled foods. You may also want to keep items such as salt, sugar, spices and hot sauces away from easy access, since using them in excess can cause an upset stomach or other health problems. In addition, consider removing items like soap, rubbing alcohol, lotions, candles or decorative "food- looking" items that may appear or smell edible to a person with Alzheimer's disease.

To help ensure safety, install good smoke detectors since your mother may not smell smoke and may not interpret the sight of smoke as danger. Also — because people with Alzheimer's disease can lose their sensation of hot and cold — adjust the water heater to 120 F to avoid scalding hot water. In addition, you may want to evaluate appliances in the home that get very hot, such as the stove, iron or coffee maker, and decide if it's safe for your loved one to use these items.

ACTION GUIDE

Health concerns

This section discusses many common health problems experienced by people with dementia, especially in later stages of the disease. This list is not a complete one. Your loved one may not experience any of the conditions described. Contact your doctor for further information on these health concerns.

Choking

As dementia progresses, your loved one may have difficulty chewing or swallowing food. Choking is often the result of inadequately chewed food becoming lodged in the throat or windpipe, blocking the passage of air. Most often, solid foods such as meat are the cause of choking.

- If food "goes down the wrong pipe," the coughing reflex often resolves the problem. A person isn't choking if he or she is able to cough freely, has normal skin color and can speak.
- A universal sign for choking is hands clutched to the throat, with thumbs and fingers extended. The person's face will assume a look of panic. He or she may wheeze or gasp and be unable to communicate except by hand motions. A person who displays these symptoms requires emergency treatment.
- Be prepared for emergencies. Ask a nurse or the Red Cross for techniques to help your loved one if he or she is choking.
- To reduce the risk of choking, serve soft, thick foods to ease the process of swallowing.
- If you mix foods in a blender, use a product called a food thickener, which is tasteless and helps to even out the texture. For example, fruit may separate into pulp and liquid, increasing the likelihood of choking. Using a thickener will smooth the texture and make swallowing easier.
- Try to make sure your loved one's head is tilted slightly forward while eating. Leaning back increases the risk of choking.

The Heimlich maneuver

This maneuver is the best known method of removing an object from the airway of a person who is choking.

1. Stand behind the choking person and wrap your arms around his or her waist. Bend the person slightly forward.
2. Make a fist with one hand and place it slightly above the person's navel.
3. Grasp your fist with the other hand and press hard into the abdomen with a quick upward thrust. Repeat this procedure until the object is expelled from the airway.

ACTION GUIDE

Dehydration

People with dementia may forget to drink enough fluids. Signs of dehydration include dry mouth, little or no urination, weakness, dizziness or lightheadedness. Dehydration also can increase confusion and cause constipation, fever and a rapid pulse.

- Encourage your loved one to drink fluids. Most healthy people meet their daily hydration needs by letting thirst be their guide, but as a caregiver for someone with dementia, you'll need to monitor fluid intake closely.
- Keep a glass of water or a favorite beverage near your loved one throughout the day. Provide gentle reminders — for example, by asking, "Is your water cold enough?"
- Drinking caffeinated beverages in moderate amounts is fine but be aware that caffeine may increase anxiety and sleeplessness. If at some point you choose to decrease your loved one's caffeine intake, phase out the caffeinated beverages gradually to reduce the risk that the symptoms of caffeine withdrawal, such as headaches, may occur.
- If your loved one was accustomed to drinking coffee throughout the day, serve noncaffeinated beverages in a coffee mug.
- If incontinence is a problem, discourage drinking fluids after the evening meal. However, don't discourage fluids altogether because of incontinence. This may cause dehydration, bladder infections and other serious complications.

Dental care

People with dementia may neglect dental hygiene and develop oral infections. Poor dental care can also affect nutrition.

- Tell your dentist about the diagnosis of dementia. Some dentists have more experience working with people with dementia than do others. Ask a support group for referrals.
- Make sure the dentist is aware of all medications the person is taking. Some medications can cause dry mouth or other conditions that could affect dental health.
- Help your loved one brush after each meal. Your dentist may be able to provide dental aids such as mouth swabs that can be used in place of a toothbrush. Ask your dentist for suggestions if your loved one is refusing to open his or her mouth for cleaning.
- Give simple one-step instructions for brushing teeth: "Take the cap off the toothpaste. Good. Now squeeze the tube. Good. Now brush your top teeth."
- Brush your own teeth at the same time to model the process.
- Help your loved one grip the toothbrush by making the handle thicker. You can do this by wrapping aluminum foil around the handle or by attaching it to a plastic bicycle handlebar grip. Or try wrapping a Velcro strap around the person's hand and tucking the toothbrush inside the strap.
- If you're helping your loved one brush, use a spoon to gently pull the cheek away from gums to help you see the teeth.
- Encourage eating raw fruits and vegetables at meals. Suggest rinsing the mouth with water after meals, particularly if the person has difficulty with brushing teeth.
- Some caregivers choose to no longer have their loved ones use dentures as the disease progresses, and so they provide the person with a soft diet. A dietitian can help you meet the specific needs of your situation.
- Refusal to eat is often a clue that a person has mouth sores or poorly fitting dentures. Ask your dentist for assistance.

Falls

Studies suggest that people with Alzheimer's disease will experience at least one fall during the course of the disease. They're also twice as likely to experience a hip fracture as people their age who don't have Alzheimer's.

- Physically restraining your loved one may not prevent falls and may actually increase the likelihood of injury. Some falls may not be preventable.
- Your loved one may not remember to call for assistance whenever he or she wants to get up, even with frequent reminders. Try putting a sign on a lap tray that says, "Stay in your chair. I'll be right back."
- Have your loved one sit on the edge of the bed for a few moments before trying to stand.
- The use of bedrails is controversial. Some people believe bedrails can prevent their loved ones from rolling out of bed or from standing up and falling. However, people with Alzheimer's have been known to climb over bedrails and fall or to injure themselves after becoming stuck between the rails. Your state may have guidelines about bedrail use.
- In case of a fall, try to remain calm. Sit with your loved one to determine if an injury has occurred. Look for signs of redness, swelling, bruises or broken bones. If you believe a bone is broken or a head injury has occurred, call for emergency medical assistance. If your loved one seems uninjured, eventually encourage the person to stand independently rather than trying to lift him or her.
- If you do try to lift your loved one, put your hands in the armpits and use your legs, rather than your back, for strength. Try to have a neighbor or family member you can call on for assistance. Remember that you'll not be able to care for your loved one if you become injured.
- A physical therapist can help determine whether your loved one could benefit from the use of a walker or other device.

Hospitalization

Hospitalization may be necessary for certain conditions, but an overnight stay can be very disruptive for a person with dementia. Find out whether care can be provided on an outpatient basis or at home instead of a hospital stay.

- If hospitalization is unavoidable, speak to the staff members about the current stage of your loved one's condition. This may be helpful if some of the staff is unfamiliar with the nature of dementia. Express your loved one's needs but try not to overwhelm the staff with too many demands. A written list of important information may prove helpful.
- Try to have family or friends on call to reassure your loved one and answer questions from the staff at times when you may not be available to do so. You need to give yourself breaks and take care of yourself, too.
- See if a private room at the hospital is an option. Bring familiar items to the room, such as pictures of family and favorite quiet music.
- You may need to ask for the services of a social worker who can help answer your questions, be your loved one's advocate and plan for discharge. Social workers are trained to help you communicate with the hospital staff and maneuver the various professional networks involved in caregiving.
- Check with the doctor frequently about how long your loved one may be expected to stay in the hospital. If you receive conflicting information from various doctors and nurses on the discharge date, ask your social worker to help you clarify the information.
- Make sure you communicate with the hospital staff about your goals for care, quality of life and pain management.

Surgery and medical treatment

When your loved one has received a diagnosis of dementia, it may be difficult deciding whether to treat other conditions that require certain interventions, such as heart surgery or chemotherapy. Here are some considerations:

- Specialists in a particular field of medicine, such as cardiology or cancer, may recommend treatments for the conditions they know best. When an invasive treatment is recommended, you also may want to discuss other options with a general practitioner or neurologist.
- General anesthesia, which is used to render a person unconscious during surgery, usually makes cognitive impairment worse. Sometimes people bounce back from the decline, but often this isn't the case. Ask your doctor if local anesthesia is possible instead.
- Ask the following questions of the specialist to help you make a well-informed decision:
  - What is the goal of treatment?
  - What benefits could treatment provide?
  - Would treatment affect the person's cognitive skills?
  - How may treatment affect the person's quality of life?
  - Is the person likely to experience pain or nausea from treatment?
  - How frightening or confusing might treatment be for the person?
- Responses to these questions may help you weigh the pros and cons of treatment. Consider your caregiving goals. Do you want to lengthen the person's life at the risk of decreasing his or her quality of life? For example, electroconvulsive therapy (ECT) for depression may impair your loved one's memory, but his or her quality of life may improve. Surgery may lengthen the person's life but decrease quality of life because of pain or diminished cognitive skills from anesthesia.

ACTION GUIDE

Medications

Your loved one may be taking medications for more than one condition at different times throughout the day. Here are suggestions to keep your loved one on track:

- Keep an updated list of medications, along with dosages and times, posted inside a cupboard door. Carry a list with you whenever you leave the house.
- Place the phone number for your doctor's office and poison control next to the phone in case of an accidental overdose.
- Use a pillbox to help keep track of medications.
- If your loved one lives alone, you may need to provide a reminder phone call and stay on the phone to ensure that the person takes the medications.
- When a new medication is prescribed, ask your doctor or nurse to provide the following information: drug name, purpose, dosage, time of day given, and potential side effects.
- If your loved one experiences changes in behavior, demeanor or physical condition, consider whether any medications have been changed recently. Contact your doctor with concerns.
- Make sure every doctor and specialist who examines your loved one is aware of all medications, especially herbal supplements and other over-the-counter products. These substances may interact with prescribed medications and cause harmful side effects.
- Don't change dosages without the consent of your physician.
- Throw out old prescriptions, and don't use medications for anyone other than the person for whom they're prescribed.
- If your loved one refuses a medication or spits it out, provide a simple explanation for its purpose. For example, "Mom, the doctor says you need to take blood pressure medication for your heart." If she continues to refuse, ask your doctor if you can crush the medication and hide it in food or juice. You may be able to obtain it in liquid form.
- Medications used to control challenging behaviors can have particularly harmful side effects. You may want to try using nonmedication interventions first.

Pain

Although dementia may not cause pain, your loved one still can experience stomach cramps, pressure sores and sprains. Problems arise as your loved one loses the ability to understand why something hurts and to tell you when something is wrong.

- Watch facial expressions and body language for signs of pain. Wincing, grimacing, tugging at clothes or pulling away from touch may indicate that your loved one is uncomfortable.
- The person may be unable to indicate where pain is occurring. Use bathing and dressing times to look for swelling, redness, bruising and other signs of inflammation or injury.
- Complaints of pain may indicate emotional distress — such as depression, boredom or fatigue — rather than physical harm.
- If pain is experienced frequently, talk to your doctor about a pain management regime that is safe for your loved one.

Pressure sores

Pressure sores may develop if your loved one sits or lies in the same position for several hours at a time. Bones wear away at muscle and skin when the body isn't regularly readjusted.

- A warning sign of pressure sores is red and swollen skin, particularly at places where the body is in contact with the chair or bed. Common locations include knees, elbows, hips, heels, shoulder blades, spine, buttocks and ankles. Eventually the red areas become open sores if not treated.
- If your loved one is sedentary, reposition him or her every two hours. Place pillows between the knees and ankles when the person is lying on his or her side. Use foam or gel pads to cushion vulnerable areas.
- A home health agency can help you provide personal care and move your loved one. Ask nursing home staff how often your loved one is repositioned throughout the day and night.
- Ill-fitting clothes can put people at risk for pressure sores. Make sure clothes are comfortable and adequate in size.

ACTION GUIDE

Sleep disturbance

Disrupted sleep patterns are common in people with dementia. Sleep disturbances may be caused by the dementia itself or by other illnesses, medications or a poorly adapted environment. Be careful of sleep medications, which may only make confusion worse. If your loved one is having difficulty sleeping, consider one of the following strategies:

- Try to maintain a regular bedtime in the daily routine.
- To indicate to your loved one that it's bedtime, yawn and stretch. Turn off the lights together as a bedtime ritual.
- Avoid discussing tomorrow's plans before bedtime. People with dementia often confuse time and start to worry.
- Avoid loud, stimulating television before bedtime. Instead, try reading aloud, playing soft music or offering a light snack to help calm your loved one.
- Have your loved one use the bathroom before bedtime.
- If changing into pajamas is upsetting for your loved one, use a cotton sweatsuit that can be worn day and night.
- Allow your loved one to sleep wherever he or she prefers, including a recliner chair or couch.
- Give the person an activity to do at night if sleep seems unlikely.
- Avoid giving the person alcohol or caffeine, especially late in the day. But be aware that quitting caffeine abruptly can cause headaches and irritability.
- Encourage your loved one to exercise regularly to burn off excess emotions.
- If background noise is keeping your loved one awake, try a white-noise generator that creates a quiet hum to counteract the noise.
- Don't discourage napping during the day, especially if it's the only sleep your loved one gets. It's better to get a little sleep rather than get no sleep at all.
- Excessive sleep is generally not a problem unless it's caused by depression, boredom or medications.

Bladder and bowel conditions

Urinary tract infection

A urinary tract infection (UTI) occurs when bacteria take hold in the bladder or the urethra — the tube that transports urine from the bladder — and multiply into a full-blown infection. Under normal circumstances, these bacteria are flushed out during urination or controlled by the antibacterial properties of urine.

- Signs and symptoms of a UTI may include frequent or urgent urination, burning pain during urination, blood or pus in the urine, and fever.
- Consider the possibility of a UTI if your loved one experiences a sudden change of behavior, such as increased anger or drowsiness, as well as increased confusion and fatigue.
- In late-stage Alzheimer's disease, UTIs are a leading cause of death. This is because the body is unable to fight off infection when the person becomes bedridden.
- If you suspect your loved one has a UTI, your doctor can perform a urinalysis and treat the infection with antibiotics.

Constipation

Constipation occurs when a person has uncharacteristically infrequent bowel movements or difficulty passing stools. Your loved one may become constipated as the effects of dementia make him or her more sedentary and immobile. Avoiding constipation is important in preventing bowel obstruction, pain and fatigue — which only increase confusion.

- A person with dementia often isn't able to keep track of bowel movements, even if he or she is in the early stages of the disease. Pain, bloating or gas may be signs of constipation.
- Help your loved one eat a balanced diet with high-fiber foods such as vegetables, fruits and whole-grain products.
- Encourage your loved one to drink plenty of fluids.
- Establish a daily routine for your loved one to attempt bowel elimination.
- The use of laxatives is generally not recommended for relieving constipation in a person with dementia.

The final stages of Alzheimer's disease

Sometimes it's difficult to know when someone is experiencing the symptoms of late-stage dementia. Generally, the person will be bedridden, no longer able to walk, and totally dependent on caregivers in all activities of daily living. Other changes may include:

- Loss of weight
- Disinterest in eating or refusal to eat
- Loss of bowel and bladder control
- Sleepiness
- Being mute or difficult to understand
- Groaning, mumbling loudly or crying out when touched
- Inability to recognize family, friends, caregivers and self
- Seizures and frequent infections

You'll face complex care decisions at this time. It's important to follow your loved one's wishes, if these are known from an advance directive. If no specific directions are known, depend on your knowledge of the person's values and beliefs for guidance.

You'll also need to consider the progress of the disease, the overall health of the person, and the risks or benefits that may be obtained from certain procedures or medications. In the late stages of dementia, options for end-of-life care generally include:

- Treatment to prolong life using all available resources, such as tube feeding for nutrition
- Treatment to maintain health, such as blood pressure medication for hypertension and insulin for diabetes
- Treatment intended to provide comfort (palliative care), primarily pain control and emotional support

Whatever you decide, you want to maintain the dignity and privacy of your loved one. Advice from your doctor, other specialists and members of a hospice team are important at this time.

You may wonder if your loved one is aware of what's going on around him or her in this last stage of the illness. Although the body and mind are in the process of shutting down, your loved one still may be aware of your care and affection. Hold hands. Stroke his or her forehead. Say what you need to say to bring closure to your relationship.

The process of grief

Grief can be defined as the process of adjusting to loss. Grief brings about intense feelings and emotions. For some, the grieving process begins long before death occurs.

The grieving process is a gradual one. Don't try to avoid the process or to simply "wait it out." You must grieve in order to bring about emotional healing and adjust to your new life situation.

- Don't try to rush through the grieving process. Remember that most people need at least two years to begin feeling "normal" after a death.
- Be open with others about what you're experiencing. Your family and friends may avoid the topic, believing this will be easier on you.
- Avoid making major decisions for at least one year.
- Follow your normal routine as much as possible, but let others help you with daily tasks. People will want to help, but they may not know how.
- Try to confront the reminders of your loved one. Notice situations when you would expect to see your loved one, and try to remind yourself of his or her death at those times.
- Identify the source of any anger and find ways to cope with it. This may mean directing your anger into something constructive such as volunteer work. Physical activity often helps release anger.
- Expect to have feelings of relief now that the responsibility of caregiving is gone.
- Try to have a realistic view of past actions and present emotions to reduce any guilt you may feel. Don't focus on what you wish you had done differently.
- Accept fear as a normal part of the grieving process. Remaining involved socially rather than isolating yourself helps assuage fear.

In this final stage of the grieving process, you quit focusing on the past and seeking an explanation for death. Instead, you begin concentrating on living life to the fullest in spite of death and looking for ways to grow from the experience.

Additional resources

AARP

601 E Street N.W.
Washington, DC 20049
888-687-2277
www.aarp.org

Administration on Aging (AOA)

330 Independence Ave. S.W.
Washington, DC 20201
202-619-0724
www.aoa.gov

Agency for Healthcare Research and Quality

Office of Communications and Knowledge Transfer
540 Gaither Road, Suite 2000
Rockville, MD 20850
301-427-1364
www.ahcpr.gov

Alzheimer's Association

National Office
225 N. Michigan Ave., Floor 17
Chicago, IL 60601
800-272-3900
www.alz.org

Alzheimer's Disease Education and Referral Center (ADEAR)

P.O. Box 8250
Silver Spring, MD 20907-8250
800-438-4380
www.alzheimers.org/adear

Alzheimer's Disease International

64 Great Suffolk Street
London SE1 0BL
United Kingdom
44-20-79810880
www.alz.co.uk

American Health Assistance Foundation

22512 Gateway Center Drive
Clarksburg, MD 20871
301-948-3244 or 800-437-2423
www.ahaf.org

Center for Drug Evaluation and Research

Food and Drug Administration
888-463-6332
www.fda.gov/cder/

Centers for Medicare and Medicaid Services

7500 Security Blvd.
Baltimore, MD 21244-1850
410-786-3000 or 877-267-2323
www.cms.hhs.gov

CenterWatch Clinical Trials Listing Service

22 Thomson Place, 47F1
Boston, MA 02210-1212
617-856-5900
www.centerwatch.com

Eldercare Locator

(Administered by the Administration on Aging)
800-677-1116
www.eldercare.gov

Family Caregiver Alliance

180 Montgomery St., Suite 1100
San Francisco, CA 94104
415-434 –3388 or 800-445-8106
www.caregiver.org

National Association of Area Agencies on Aging

1730 Rhode Island Ave., NW, Suite 1200
Washington, DC 20036
202-872-0888
www.n4a.org

National Association of State Units on Aging

1201 15th Street N.W., Suite 350
Washington, DC 20005
202-898-2578
www.nasua.org

National Council on the Aging

300 D Street, S.W., Suite 801
Washington, DC 20024
202-479-1200
www.ncoa.org

National Hospice and Palliative Care Organization

1700 Diagonal Road, Suite 625
Alexandria, VA 22314
703-837-1500
www.nhpco.org

National Institute of Mental Health (NIMH)

Public Information and Communications Branch
6001 Executive Blvd., Room 8184, MSC 9663
Bethesda, MD 20892-9663
301-443-4513 or 866-615-6464
www.nimh.nih.gov

National Institute of Neurological Disorders and Stroke

P.O. Box 5801
Bethesda, MD 20824
301-496-5751 or 800-352-9424
www.ninds.nih.gov

National Institutes of Health Clinical Center

800-411-1222
www.cc.nih.gov

National Institute on Aging

Building 31, Room 5C27
31 Center Drive, MSC 2292
Bethesda, MD 20892
301-496-1752
www.nia.nih.gov

National Library of Medicine

8600 Rockville Pike
Bethesda, MD 20894
888-346-3656
www.nlm.nih.gov

Society for Neuroscience

11 Dupont Circle N.W., Suite 500
Washington, DC 20036
202-462-6688
www.sfn.org

Index

MRI scans — cont.
  in brain shrinkage diagnosis,
      60–61
  in brain structure/activity
      changes, 56–57
  in CJD diagnosis, 161
  diffusion-weighted, 208
  in FTD diagnosis, 53, 125
  functional (fMRI), 50, 209
  in hippocampus
      measurement, 207–208
  in Huntington's disease
      diagnosis, 157
  in MCI diagnosis, 179
  in VCI diagnosis, 53, 148
  See also brain imaging
MS (multiple sclerosis), 167–169
  signs and symptoms, 168
  symptom and severity,
      168–169
  treatment, 169
multiple sclerosis. *See* MS
muscle coordination, loss of, 43
muscular changes, 24
myelin, 30

N

Namenda. *See* memantine
neurodegenerative disorders,
      9–10
neurofibrillary tangles.
      See tangles
neurological evaluation, 46
neurons
  in cell communication, 30–31
  defined, 29
  function, 29
  loss, 66
  plaques, 58, 82, 83, 201–202
  structure illustration, 30

neuropsychological tests, 178
  common, 47
  function, 46–47, 48
  results, 47
neurotransmitter levels, 67
non-amnestic MCI, 175
  causes, 177
  defined, 175
  See also mild cognitive
      impairment (MCI)
non-steroidal anti-inflammatory
      drugs (NSAIDs), 183, 212
normal aging, 20, 22
  cardiovascular changes,
      23–24
  cognitive changes, 33–35
  metabolism changes, 24–25
  physical changes with, 21–25
  sensory changes, 24
  skeletal/muscular changes,
      24
  See also aging
normal pressure hydrocephalus,
      14, 154–156
  illustrated, 154
  signs and symptoms, 155
  treatment, 155–156
nortriptyline, 158
nursing homes, 297
nutritional deficiencies, as
      dementia cause, 14
nutritional support, 127

O

occipital lobe, 27
olanzapine, 139
organization(memory), 187-188
oxidative stress, 87
  beta-amyloid fragments, 88
  vitamin E for, 102–103